GYM-FREE
and RIPPED

Weight-Free Workouts
That Build and Sculpt

Nathan Jendrick

ALPHA

A member of Penguin Group (USA) Inc.

ALPHA BOOKS

Published by the Penguin Group

Penguin Group (USA) Inc., 375 Hudson Street, New York, New York 10014, USA

Penguin Group (Canada), 90 Eglinton Avenue East, Suite 700, Toronto, Ontario M4P 2Y3, Canada (a division of Pearson Penguin Canada Inc.)

Penguin Books Ltd., 80 Strand, London WC2R 0RL, England

Penguin Ireland, 25 St. Stephen's Green, Dublin 2, Ireland (a division of Penguin Books Ltd.)

Penguin Group (Australia), 250 Camberwell Road, Camberwell, Victoria 3124, Australia (a division of Pearson Australia Group Pty. Ltd.)

Penguin Books India Pvt. Ltd., 11 Community Centre, Panchsheel Park, New Delhi—110 017, India

Penguin Group (NZ), 67 Apollo Drive, Rosedale, North Shore, Auckland 1311, New Zealand (a division of Pearson New Zealand Ltd.)

Penguin Books (South Africa) (Pty.) Ltd., 24 Sturdee Avenue, Rosebank, Johannesburg 2196, South Africa

Penguin Books Ltd., Registered Offices: 80 Strand, London WC2R 0RL, England

International Standard Book Number: 978-1-61564-099-7
Library of Congress Catalog Card Number: 2011901231

13   12   11   8   7   6   5   4   3   2   1

Interpretation of the printing code: The rightmost number of the first series of numbers is the year of the book's printing; the rightmost number of the second series of numbers is the number of the book's printing. For example, a printing code of 11-1 shows that the first printing occurred in 2011.

Printed in the United States of America

Publisher: *Marie Butler-Knight*
Associate Publisher: *Mike Sanders*
Executive Managing Editor: *Billy Fields*
Acquisitions Editor: *Tom Stevens*
Development Editor: *Jennifer Moore*
Senior Production Editor: *Janette Lynn*
Copy Editor: *Daron Thayer*

Cover Designer: *Rebecca Batchelor*
Book Designer: *Rebecca Batchelor*
Indexer: *Tonya Heard*
Layout: *Rebecca Batchelor, Ayanna Lacey*
Proofreader: *John Etchison*
Photos: *Nathan Jendrick*

"I do it as a therapy. I do it as something to keep me alive. We all need a little discipline. Exercise is my discipline."

—In memory of Jack LaLanne (1914–2011), who deserves unending recognition for inspiring millions, and for carrying on the best conversations about health and fitness that I have ever had.

Contents

Introduction

Gym-Free and Ripped is more than a fitness guide, it's a lifestyle. Through effective exercise, proper nutrition, and clear mental focus, *being* gym-free and ripped is knowing that anywhere you go, no matter what you are doing, you are in control of your life. As a healthy, happy, and energetic individual, you're living life to the fullest and bettering yourself each and every day. You don't have to join a health club, hire a personal trainer, or follow the latest diet trend. Instead, the gym-free lifestyle requires only a little time, a lot of desire, and a goal of leaving the normal behind and becoming an extraordinary example of health and happiness.

The ultimate goal of this book—this compilation of information—is to give you all of the tools necessary to take control of your own personal well-being. Make no mistake, changing bad habits and creating healthy new ones can be a daunting task. And that type of struggle doesn't even have to have anything to do with fitness. When it comes to training, exercise, and proper nutrition, you have the media and countless companies around the world further confusing your efforts by trying to pitch you a new fad diet or a "miracle" pill that will supposedly solve all of your ailments seamlessly. But, as you've shown you know by picking up a book that doesn't have the words "Miracle" or "Instant" on the cover, making lifelong changes takes work and takes time. However, those changes that are made with quality knowledge and at an appropriate pace are changes that will last a lifetime. Fad diets are as lasting as their names and a pill is useful for no longer than it takes to pass through your system. Thus, by picking up something that will *teach* you how to control your own body, you're doing yourself—and everyone who cares about you—a great service.

Along with providing you with the information necessary to get you into the best shape of your life—and being able to achieve that and maintain it anywhere—this book is aimed to rid you of that mindless nonsense proliferating too many TV commercials and fitness magazines. To truly believe in what you're doing and to really understand that *you* are truly in control, you've got to understand the whys and the hows of every step. Anyone can follow a high-priced personal trainer around the gym and go through the motions, and you just might get into decent shape by doing this. But if all you're doing is following and listening (and paying the hefty bill), you're not actually learning anything. As soon as you stop opening your wallet for that hourly rate, you're left in the proverbial ocean without a life jacket. So to ensure that you will always be in position to be your best, I will explain all of the life-changing steps contained in this book to you. And this education will include a lot of myth busting, so the next time your friend says, "So on the radio I heard …", you can help them out by saving time, frustration, and potentially a lot of money.

Preventing the "I wish I had known …" Reflection

People often take continuing education classes, surf the Internet, and read all kinds of reference materials to learn new skills or learn about things that interest them. For some reason, though, this often does not extend to health and fitness! It likely has something to do with the proliferation of the previously mentioned fad diets, pills, and personal trainers. As such, when people finally do get to the point of controlling their own routine, they start back at square one and become a student again—at a point where they should be in the driver's seat again, so to speak. Everyone has been there, it's profoundly common. At one point or another, every fit person can look back and say, "I wish I had known …." While you can't get back time previously spent, another goal of *Gym-Free and Ripped* is to prevent any more of those kinds of personal reflections. And because so many of the most important facts are also the most basic, I'm going to start with that right now. Here are a few things that you should understand right away, which will also be covered more throughout the book:

1. There is no magic pill!

While it will be covered significantly more in Chapter 8, you need to know right out of the gate that there is no magic pill for fitness. Even some of the "best" thermogenic "fat burners" on the market may only increase your metabolism by 50 or so calories a day. That's about half of a banana! And at upwards of $60 a bottle, you're better off saving your cash and going for a slow half-mile walk that, conveniently enough, also burns about 50 calories. So while some supplements can be quite beneficial, remember that they're *supplementary*. They can't do the real work for you, and a large number of products you see on store shelves should be avoided.

2. No Amount of Quality Training Fixes Poor Nutrition

You can go for all of the runs you want and lift all of the weights you want, but if you don't give your body the proper fuel, you're not going to see results. Some diets that have had their 15 minutes of fame try saying you can eat anything you want as long as you do their very specific program. When you don't get the body you're after, surely the blame is placed on you not matching their pace, reps, or weights exactly as the guy on TV had written it. The truth is much simpler: junk in, junk out. If you're putting bad stuff into your program, don't expect to get good stuff out of it, no matter how much you throw into it. You wouldn't expect any kind of seed to grow big and healthy if you put it into hard, dirty, and contaminated soil, so don't expect anything different of yourself.

People look at fitness as 90 percent training, 10 percent nutrition. While there's no perfect ratio because everyone's body is so different, you're nonetheless going to be much closer if you reverse those numbers.

3. Weight Doesn't Matter

A huge mistake for people who are training, whether they're new to it or have years invested, is that they're too focused on weight—whether it's the weight being lifted or weight on the scale. The fact is, neither one matters. The weight you lift need only be enough to stimulate your muscles. As you'll learn throughout these pages, you can do that with just the bodyweight you already have. And if you want to add variety or increase tension, you can use very simple materials to do that. No gym or stack of iron plates is required. As for the weight on the scale, what it reads makes no difference. What really matters is how you look and feel. Remember, if you lose body fat and add muscle mass, your weight may not change (it might even go up), but you'll look like a whole different person.

4. "Superheroes" Often Have "Special" Help

The number of people, young and old, who see guys on magazine covers or in action movies and say, "I want to look like that!" grows every day. Everyone has their goals and their desires and they should all be supported. With that said, it's unfair for companies to promote that certain physique types are obtainable without pharmaceutical help. While these larger-than-life body types sell show tickets and movie passes, all too often they're also used to sell protein and multi-vitamins. Unfortunately, no matter how many trips you take to vitamin and supplement stores, you won't find the things that some open-class professional bodybuilders use to carry that much muscle mass. That's not to demonize anyone's personal choice on what they put into their own body. However, because it can cause people frustration to the point that they quit exercising when they don't see the same progress, it's worth noting what is realistic and what takes anabolic steroids to achieve. So while you might see your favorite superhero on the movie screen looking ripped, you might also see him on the nightly news with some legal problems pertaining to certain drugs found in his luggage.

Everyone has a different level of genetic potential when it comes to carrying a certain amount of muscle. Embrace yours and make yourself the absolute best you can be. This journey into better health is all about *you*—don't compare yourself to anyone else!

Acknowledgments

My greatest amount of gratitude goes out to my family for their support: Don Anderson and Christena Warwick, Michael Jendrick, and my parents, Tom and Janice Tani. The appreciation I have for my parents who assured me that I didn't have to stay that overweight, inactive, and unhappy teenager that I was simply cannot be overstated.

I also offer many thanks to everyone involved in the creation of this book from the very beginning to the very end: to my agent Marilyn Allen, to Tom Stevens, Janette Lynn, and the entire Alpha Books team, and to Jennifer Moore. Infinite appreciation also goes out to an absolutely inspiring athlete and person, Rich Roll, and to my friend and NGA Professional Bodybuilder, Paul "Peanut" Tomko.

Finally, my unending love to my wife, Megan Jendrick, and to our first baby who we just learned to expect during the editing period of this book. You both make me want to always be better in absolutely every way a man can be.

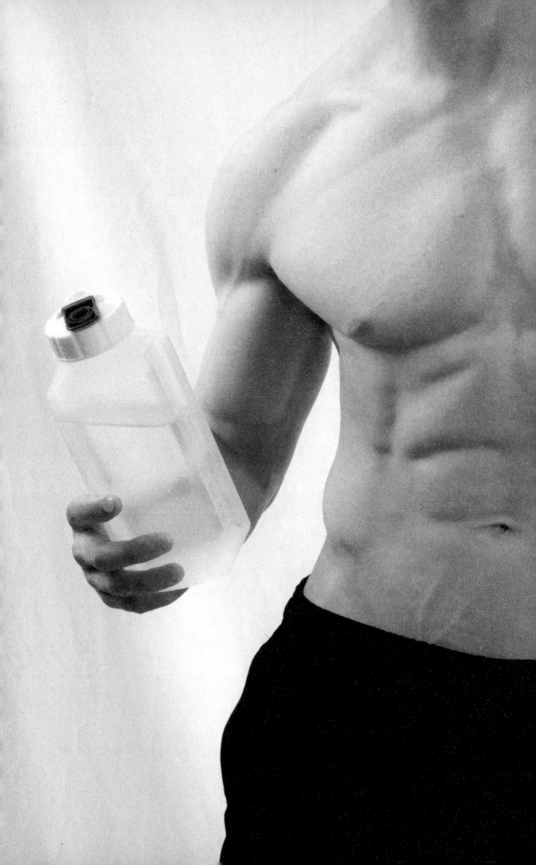

1

The Gym-Free Method

The gym-free method is a mind-set and a way of life. With it, you don't need a gym to have the body of your dreams, and you don't need fancy machines with televisions and fans installed in them to improve your health. Furthermore, you don't have to give up an entire class of nutrients—whether carbs or fats—to burn body fat. The gym-free mind-set is knowing that being healthy is a lifestyle, not a fad, and it isn't something you check in or out of with swipes of a membership card.

For too long, the media and salesmen have made the rules about what fitness requires: Fancy—and expensive—home machines that take up too much space and deliver too little. Miracle pills and potions that taste horrible and do no good. Gadgets that put your body in such awkward positions even gymnasts wouldn't be comfortable using them. These products don't get you any closer to fitness, only closer to frustration. When logic prevails, the truth is revealed: People are designed to be fit using nothing but their bodies.

Think about those who defend our country in the military. Think about Olympic champions who succeed on fields, on tracks, and in pools around the world. The vast majority of these people train and prepare to do great things simply with their bodies. No Bowflex, no Total-Gym, no Ab-Roller, and certainly no gym membership. Those who succeed without excessive intervention through mechanical means embody the gym-free mind-set. And for you, this isn't about winning Olympic medals, it's about something much more important: your health. And every day that passes in which you aren't focused on getting fit, you're missing a great opportunity to feel and look better for the rest of your life. Don't follow the crowd and sit around and do nothing; get up, get active, and get *ripped.*

America is becoming a nation of fatties. Reports tell us by 2020 more than 75 percent of Americans will be overweight, which would make us the fattest country on record, a rather dubious honor. Yet, in the face of these facts, most people lack the desire to take a stand and make a change. By picking up this book, you are setting yourself apart from the crowd, and taking the first of many steps on a journey to a healthier you, and thus, a healthier "us."

The biggest part of developing a "new you" is finding the strength within yourself to create the positive changes you have always dreamed of. You have to find it within yourself to dedicate your actions to doing what it takes to get what you want. It's an effort-to-reward balance that's different for every person, and something only you hold the key to. Your life is different than anyone else's, your schedule is different, and your goals are different. But like anyone else, once you figure out what it is you really want, there is no one to stop you but yourself.

This book isn't just about showing you the right exercises to do to develop the body you've always wanted, nor is it about just showing you the best-tasting healthy foods. This book is welcoming you to an entire program for people who are busy, always on the go, but goal-oriented and determined to better their health and their lives mentally and physically.

Get Ready for Results

The first step in starting a new health routine is getting your mind into it. The physical portion of training is easy. No matter how hard it feels at first, you'll find in very little time that your body is stronger than you ever thought. You'll learn after just your first few workouts that, upon reflection, it was your mind giving up and not your body. The human body is an amazingly resilient work of art that is limited by the mind that runs it. So to get the most out of it, you have to prepare yourself mentally to achieve results physically.

Mentally Preparing for the New You

Getting yourself mentally prepared involves coming to terms with the following key concepts:

- Getting fit will take some adjustments in your schedule.

- You'll be eating differently than most of your friends.

- You'll have to endure a certain level of sacrifice.

Getting fit is like anything else worth doing: it takes effort and sacrifice, and it involves changes. But know, too, that it's all worth it, it's all for your own betterment, and it's all immensely rewarding.

As for when to start your new routine, it is always a good idea to familiarize yourself with the program before starting. That isn't to say you need to read this book from cover to cover before beginning, but I do encourage you to flip through and read bits here and there to get acquainted with the material. Just like studying in school, it's good to go over the text before taking the exam. The main difference is this exam—testing your limits and grading your progress—is a lot more fun and rewarding.

And here is something that goes against conventional wisdom: if you have a vacation coming up in a few days or a week, don't worry about hitting the full program straightaway. Get started, get your body moving, and when you return from your trip you can fully invest yourself. The television infomercials will tell you that you need to start *now!* if you want to succeed, but they don't take into account the real world. If you're worried about following a strict new diet that you don't quite have down yet while you're supposed to be enjoying sunshine and sand, you can't really enjoy your vacation. You'll waste the money you spent setting it up and, ultimately, you'll start thinking about what your fitness program has cost you rather than helped you gain. The mental strength to change your life is a huge aspect of staying mentally strong and working things out for *you.*

You can start *now.* You don't have to immediately make every change outlined in this book. Take baby steps if you need to, don't overwhelm yourself, don't stress yourself out trying to make a complete 180-degree change in your lifestyle. Start small, and you will indeed make that complete turnaround. The people who do this successfully—those who change their lives and maintain their healthy habits and new, fit bodies—are those who take it slow and do it right.

So pick a date on the calendar, wrap your head around it, smile, and get yourself determined and excited for the great things heading your way.

Physically Preparing for the New You

Once you're mentally ready, the rest is simple. Physically preparing isn't really so much a preface as it is part of the program. The thing that is important to remember here is that everyone is different. You may see things in this book that are currently beyond your abilities. That's okay. It is perfectly acceptable to adjust to what suits your physical condition in the here and now. If you aren't able to do an exercise right away, then set a goal (and we will talk a lot about goals as we go) to get yourself to the point where you can complete it within a certain time period.

When it comes to training, you'll find that you are the most sore when you first start. This is when you have to be the most disciplined about sticking with the program. Your body has to train properly to get past that point, and your mind has to be tough enough to make sure you keep coming back. But as you continue to work out, you will find the discomfort is significantly reduced and, when the natural chemicals in the brain release as a result of quality exercise, you'll begin to feel fantastic when you push yourself.

Depending on your current level of fitness, you may find it beneficial to do some easy walking or other light exercise for a few days before delving into the exercises described here. If you've been away from training for a while or have been sedentary for one reason or another, give yourself a few days of lighter movement to just get your mind and body warmed up.

And, of course, because nothing is one size fits all, if you find that you start too strenuously right off the bat, you can always dial it down to what suits you. Do what's challenging yet comfortable, and never push yourself to the point of actual pain. You will soon discover there's a type of "good" pain that comes from training hard, but always avoid the discomfort that you know just isn't right.

Why Train?

I don't expect you to just take my word for how beneficial this training thing really is for you. Numerous doctors and scientific research backs up everything I say about the benefits of exercise.

Science Chimes in on the Benefits

In 2007, the *Journal of Bone and Mineral Research* released a study showing that individuals who exercise when young can incur lifelong benefits in terms of bone structure and strength and potentially reduce risk of fractures later in life, when they are most prevalent.

The Obesity Society, a group dedicated to studying and encouraging research on the causes and treatments of obesity, found that the simple act of walking combined with some healthy dietary adjustments can improve body composition. In a study released in 2007, the group found that walking for even less than an hour a day suppresses appetite, reduces stress, and causes notable (up to 10% of body weight) weight loss.

In 2008, the Mayo Clinic released a list of benefits associated with just a half-hour of exercise daily. They included a reduction of LDL cholesterol (the bad kind), an increase in HDL cholesterol (the good kind), a lowered risk of type-2 diabetes, lower blood pressure, lower risk for cancer and heart disease, and an improvement in bone density.

Can't sleep? The American Academy of Sleep Medicine showed in a 2008 study how aerobic exercise reduces anxiety and improves the quality of sleep in patients suffering from insomnia.

Improving Mental Health

As if improving your health and the way you look isn't enough to make you feel good, exercise actually improves your mental health. According to the Mayo Clinic, when you exercise you release a variety of chemicals in the brain that make you happier, more relaxed, and less stressed, and increase your self-esteem and confidence. Not bad for just getting up and moving around. You already know that exercise promotes better, more restful sleep. And the benefits from better rest? Improved concentration and productivity, a more enjoyable sex life, and elevated and improved mood, among other things.

And because aging is a fact of life for everyone, this bit of information may be particularly insightful: a 2010 published study by the American Academy of Neurology found that walking at least 6 miles a week preserves brain size and, ultimately, may help preserve memory in old age.

Now, again, if you listen to the people on your television, you'll need a gym or fancy home equipment to make all of this happen. Let me reiterate: you absolutely do not need a gym or any fancy equipment. Not only can you get the body of your dreams and the health you deserve right from home, but you can save a lot of money, too. Let's take a look.

Cost Comparisons

Let's do a cost comparison over three types of training. We'll compare training with pure body weight exercises from home, training with the optional accessories covered in this book—which we'll call "enhanced" training—and the traditional gym.

Five-Year Costs for Pure Body Weight Exercises:	
Initial cost:	$0
Cumulative cost after one year:	$0
Cumulative cost after three years:	$0
Cumulative cost after five years:	$0
Total cost	**$0**

Working out at home with no additional accessories doesn't cost a dime. You don't have any equipment costs, gym fees, or transportation costs.

Five-Year Costs for Enhanced Training (Body Weight plus Accessories)	
Initial cost:	$380
Adjustable dumbbell set	$250
BOSU Ball	$99
Exercise Ball	$20
Stretch Cord	$11
Cumulative cost after one year:	$380
Cumulative cost after three years	$380
Cumulative cost after five years	$380
Total cost	**$380**

Depending on how much weight you want, adjustable dumbbell sets range from $70 up to $400. For this estimate, we used an amount somewhere near the middle. Once you've made your initial investment in equipment, your annual costs are zero. You don't have to pay any gym fees or cover transportation costs for getting to and from the gym.

Five-Year Costs for Gym Training	
Initial cost	$100 initiation fee
Cumulative cost after one year	$1,228
Cumulative cost after three years	$3,484
Cumulative cost after five years	**$5,740**

A majority of gyms charge an "initiation fee" between $50 and $150. For this exercise, we estimated with the median of $100. We also assumed you already had clothes that are comfortable wearing at the gym.

The average gym in the United States charges between $40 and $50 each month for membership. Using the median of $45 per month for one year, we reach a $540 annual total. Assuming your gym isn't too far and you have a relatively fuel-efficient vehicle, let's presume that your to/from trip takes one gallon of fuel at an estimated $3/gallon. If you train three days each week, that totals $9/week. If you train four days each week, that's $12/week. If you train five, we have an expense of $15/week. Again, using our median cost, we have $12/week, which we multiply by 49 weeks a year (assuming you took a total of 3 weeks off from missed days here and there) and we reach a $588 fuel charge for the year, for a total of $1,228 per year for fees and transportation costs.

So as you can see, you're saving *big* money whether you use body movements alone or if you go with the enhanced route to add some extra variety. And that's even if you go all out and buy everything suggested, which you certainly don't have to do. Maybe you are only intrigued by one or two accessories, such as the exercise ball and stretch cord; then you're still getting increased variety and saving even more. This is a win-win situation.

And let's face it, on top of the financial incentives, training by yourself is a lot less hassle: You can wear whatever you want. You can grunt as loud as you want (if you're the grunting type). You don't have to worry about fellow gym-goers getting in your way or not cleaning up their equipment when they are done using it. Gym hours are irrelevant. Weather makes no difference. And if you like jamming to some music, the choice is yours. So let's get into setting up *your* ideal program.

The benefits from exercising regularly are vast, and the studies that prove them just keep adding up. And all of these benefits are available from wherever you are, wherever you're reading this, *right now*. So without further ado, let's get you in the program!

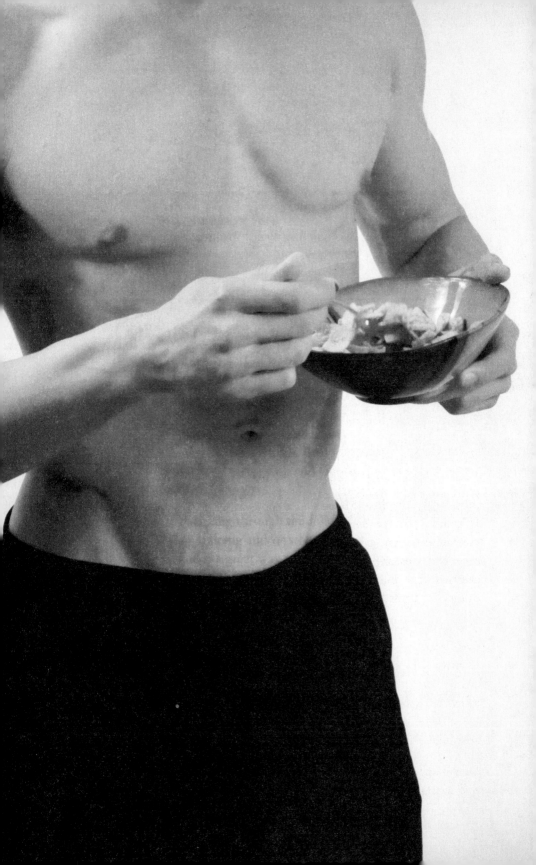

2

Eat Right to Look Great

Proper nutrition is the real key to getting in shape and getting the body you have always wanted. It doesn't matter how flashy the ads are for the latest fitness craze, the bottom line is that working out alone cannot—and will not—give you ripped abs. Life isn't that simple. You have to have the discipline to work hard not just when you train your muscles, but also with your appetite. What you put in your mouth is actually more important than what you do on the training ground. Nutrition, in fact, is the real force behind being ripped. You can be strong as an ox, but if you don't eat properly, you'll never look the way you want to. What you eat is the core of fitness and, thus, this program.

Whether you want to gain muscle or burn body fat, you have to feed yourself properly. To gain muscle you need adequate protein, quality carbohydrates, and healthy fats. To burn fat you need to decrease your caloric intake and avoid foods that spike your blood sugar or contain things like trans fats.

Part of the gym-free mind-set is being able to discern what's healthy from what's not healthy. This chapter teaches you everything you need to know to eat right at home or on the go as well as how to fuel your body with just the right amount of nutrition. You'll learn how to transform your current diet into a nutrition program designed to consistently fuel excellence by eating more often to promote satiety, and by making healthier, lower-calorie choices.

Always keep in mind that no matter how much you work out, no matter how hard you push yourself, the only way to get results is to couple that training with the right kinds—and the right amounts—of quality food. You do this by manipulating what is called your baseline diet. In fact, all of your goals—building muscle and burning fat—hinge on your baseline diet.

Establishing Your Baseline Diet

Baseline diet isn't a term you should be afraid of. It isn't any sort of fancy program like the Atkins Diet or the "Mediterranean Diet" or even the South Beach Diet. It's a simple, real-world gauge of how much you are eating, so that you can make adjustments to achieve your goals.

By definition, "baseline" simply means a reference point or starting point. It establishes something to be used in the future. For our purposes, it determines what your body is used to eating, so that you can then manipulate that information to achieve your physical goals. This is important because your body tries very hard to achieve homeostasis no matter how much you eat; if you eat more food than you need, your body will try to speed up your metabolism through increased thyroid output and other pathways to burn the energy (calories) you consume. Obviously, your body can't speed up your metabolism infinitely, and this is how body fat gets collected.

By the same token, if you suddenly cut out hundreds of calories your body has grown accustomed to, your thyroid will grind to a halt, your metabolism will slow to a snail's pace, and your body composition will not improve. This very principle is why crash diets just don't work. Sure, you may drop a few pounds right away as your body uses some fat for fuel, but once it realizes there isn't adequate nutrition reaching the stomach, you're in trouble.

The simple solution is to gradually increase the number of quality calories you consume. It's that easy. What this baseline diet does for you is give you a number your body is already familiar with; you can then divide up that number, substitute healthier foods, and make effective changes on a feasible basis. As you make these changes you're more likely to find that, because they are easy and gradual, you can maintain the results for the rest of your life. And to help, you'll find a host of healthy recipes in Appendix B to get you going.

Counting Calories

The first step to finding your baseline calorie total is to count the calories of the foods you're used to eating. Doing so for three days will give you a solid sample, though if you have an ever-changing schedule you may want to go with a five-day log to give yourself a better average. And that's what you're looking for: the average number of calories your body is used to getting.

A general warning: don't change your habits simply because you're counting calories. It's very common for people to realize halfway through the first day of keeping a diet log how bad they've been eating and suddenly clean it up. What happens then is the first day of the log is full of McDonald's, beer, and ice cream, and the next two days are broccoli, lettuce, and water. And ultimately, the final baseline count is off by thousands of calories.

If you finish your log and you look it over and realize it's not an accurate representation of your diet, start over. You're only going to hurt yourself if you don't start off on the right foot, and there's no shame in having a log that's full of junk food if that's how you're used to eating. In fact, you'll laugh later when you look back on it and see how far you've come. So be honest with yourself and be diligent about keeping track.

Your Food Log

You'll be keeping track of four basic things in your food log. Feel free to write the following categories at the top of a piece of paper and make lines straight down to separate the boxes:

Time: Because when you eat is an important key in properly feeding the well-trained body, you'll want to know when you do the majority of your eating.

Food: This is a reminder of what you ate. "Doughnut" works, but if you'd rather put "Cinnamon Apple Filled Glazed Krispy Kreme Sugared

Doughnut," you're certainly entitled to do that, as well. Make sure you write down solid foods as well as liquids and beverages.

Size: How much did you eat? One doughnut? 16 ounces of that tasty candy bar in a cup (a.k.a. a Starbucks Frappucino)? Keeping my earlier discussion of serving sizes in mind, remember to write down the actual size of the serving you ate rather than what is listed as the serving size. A box of Wheat Thins crackers may tell you a serving is 13 crackers, but if you had 39, make sure you notate accordingly.

Calories: This is the most important part of the chart. How many calories were in that drink or food you had? Be sure you're not just taking the number that falls under serving on the label. In the Wheat Thins example, a serving of 13 crackers could be 130 calories, but if you had three servings' worth, make sure you put down 390 calories.

You may find at the end of the day you need to go back and find the caloric content of something you ate or drank; having noted how much of what you had turns this into an easy task, especially if you wrote out a more detailed description.

Here's a sample chart:

Sample Food Log

Time of Day	Food/Drink	Size/Ounces	Calories
8 A.M.	Yoplait Yogurt	1 cup	100
8 A.M.	Thomas Bagel	1 bagel	250
8 A.M.	Water	8 oz.	0
10:30 A.M.	Scrambled eggs	4 whole eggs	280
11 A.M.	Diet Coke	24 oz.	0
Day 1 Totals:	**Fluid_____**	**Calories_____**	

You can often find calorie information for foods from chain eateries and fast food restaurants such as Olive Garden, Red Lobster, Starbucks, McDonald's, Burger King, and Taco Bell, on their websites.

For food you eat at home that doesn't have a nutrition label, you can find calorie information online. Some websites that include nutrition data include caloriecount.about.com, nutritiondata.self.com, and www.calorieking.com/foods.

After you've finished your log (whether it be three or five days), take the final calorie totals for each day and add them together. Divide by the number of days, and you've got your base total. Example:

> Day 1: 3200
>
> Day 2: 3600
>
> Day 3: 2975
>
> Total: 9775
>
> Divided by 3 (rounded up): 3260

The following pages provide you three days' worth of blank food logs to get you started.

Day 1: Food Log

Time of Day	Food/Drink	Size/Ounces	Calories

Day ___ Totals: Fluid_____   Calories_____

Day 2: Food Log

Time of Day	Food/Drink	Size/Ounces	Calories

Day ___ Totals: Fluid_____   Calories_____

Day 3: Food Log

Time of Day	Food/Drink	Size/Ounces	Calories

Day ___ Totals: Fluid_____   Calories_____

Adjusting Calories for Specific Goals

Armed with your baseline diet calorie total, you're now ready to set a plan for yourself. The first thing you should do is divide your baseline calorie total into six separate meals. If six meals is difficult for you, start adding meals to your day slowly at first. If you currently eat just three or four times a day, try adding one meal every few days and adjust the breakdown as you go. Using our 3,260-calorie baseline diet as a guideline, it would look like this:

Four meals:

> Meal 1: 815 calories
>
> Meal 2: 815 calories
>
> Meal 3: 815 calories
>
> Meal 4: 815 calories

Once you're able to do that comfortably, add another meal and divide your calories out once again.

Five meals:

> Meal 1: 650 calories
>
> Meal 2: 650 calories
>
> Meal 3: 650 calories
>
> Meal 4: 650 calories
>
> Meal 5: 650 calories

After five meals become manageable, add one more.

Six meals:

> Meal 1: 540 calories
>
> Meal 2: 540 calories
>
> Meal 3: 540 calories

Meal 4: 540 calories

Meal 5: 540 calories

Meal 6: 540 calories

You'll want to spread your meals throughout the day to give your body consistent nutrition. Eating every three hours is a schedule that many people find effective, which has them eating at 7 A.M., 10 A.M., 1 P.M., 4 P.M., 7 P.M. and lastly at 10 P.M. Adjust for your schedule and make it work for you.

Now, before I continue, an infinite number of people will tell you six meals a day is ideal. But there is also an infinite number that will tell you that five is okay, or that four is just as good, or that the classic "three square meals" is as good today as it was 100 years ago. At the other end of the spectrum, I've worked with Olympic athletes who eat no fewer than *ten* meals a day. And believe it or not, despite the lack of consensus, there is research to back up whichever ideology you choose. Whether you eat three meals or six meals, science tells us you can get in great shape and be healthy following that pattern. For the gym-free program, though, I suggest multiple meals spaced out because it promotes a more consistent feeling of satisfaction. You're simply not as hungry when you eat quality foods more often; plus, you are much, much less likely to overeat at a meal. It's just like being thirsty: Wait until you're parched, and you'll chug liquid as soon as you can. But if you drink consistently, you'll get along quite well with a lot less.

With that out of the way, let's move on to the practical application of the baseline diet. You're going to notice right away that eating healthy food in the quantities to achieve the neighborhood of 3,000 calories or more can be difficult. Most people would think nothing of finishing off a McDonald's Double Quarter Pounder with Cheese Extra Value Meal (with a Coke, of course), but would scoff at the idea of eating three grilled chicken breasts, a cup of brown rice, a potato, a cup of broccoli, four eggs, a banana, and 4 ounces of seasoned ground turkey meat. Yet, the Value Meal has over 1,500 calories in one sitting while the plethora of "healthy" foods, even all combined, total hundreds of calories less.

Eating well is not only filling, but it's just as delicious. Too many people have used the excuse that they can't stick to a diet because they're hungry all the time; the simple fact is they just aren't eating the right foods.

While you're getting used to eating more often, stick with the calorie total you found through your baseline log and eat foods you're used to. After that, slowly start adjusting the compositions of your meals with suggestions made in this chapter and from those discussed throughout the remainder of the book. When you're comfortable manipulating your caloric intake, do so in the neighborhood of 250 calories or so at a time, taken or added evenly throughout your meals. If your goal is to lose body fat, start reducing the total; if you're looking to add weight, trickle in that extra food throughout the day.

New Wave Nutrition for Instant Results

With a general understanding of what makes up the food you eat and how each particular facet affects you, you'll be able to make immediate changes to your meal plans that will provide rapid results you can see and feel.

Eating for Energy

Most people maintain a basic understanding of dietary needs that goes something like this: eat less, lose weight; eat more, gain weight. Although this is partially accurate, people don't generally think of the role nutrition plays in their daily energy expenditure.

You don't just wake up and feel like you're going to jump out of bed and tackle the world. Your energy levels are highly dependent on the foods you eat and the rest you've received. If you eat fast food for weeks on end, you're going to feel sluggish, bloated, and easily fatigued. If you've been eating quality foods in the right proportions, you'll have sustained energy throughout the day. No caffeine, fat burners, or energy drinks required.

Eating to Lose Fat and Gain Muscle

At the most basic level, eating less does at least initially result in weight loss. But to ensure you get ripped, you need to understand the difference between body weight and body composition.

First piece of advice: Throw away your scale. Donate it. Give it to your neighbor. Do anything with it that involves getting it out of your home. You don't need it.

Weight is a measure of overall mass. The idea behind getting in shape is to increase lean body tissue and decrease adipose (fat) tissue. Although you won't be replacing a pound of one with a pound of the other at exactly the same rate, there's going to be a constant fluctuation. If you put on five pounds of muscle and lose five pounds of fat, you're going to look very different in the mirror, but the scale won't budge. That's not a bad thing, but people who are fixated on their weight will see this as a sign of no progress, which is ridiculous.

To take an extreme example: The top bodybuilders in the world are close to 300 pounds and, when they are in contest condition, have between 3 and 4 percent body fat. There's hardly a place on their bodies you could even pinch fat, yet they tip the scales with a weight most people would consider fat. Moral of the story: Don't worry about your weight.

Eating to lose fat is a combination of properly timing your meals, eating foods that won't spike your blood sugar (low Glycemic Index carbohydrates, which will be discussed shortly) so you aren't promoting fat storage, eating energy-rich foods that complement your workout routine, and providing adequate protein for muscle recovery. To gain muscle, you're giving your body the amino acids and building blocks it needs to put on fresh, new muscle tissue and allowing yourself to take in adequate calories to support the process. It isn't rocket science, it just takes focus, discipline, and hard work.

Healthy Meal Planning Decisions

You're always going to have choices. Whether it's eating out or making something at home, or deciding between white bread and whole wheat bread, you should be cognizant of your options. Making the right choices will go a long way to achieving a healthier you.

Good protein choices: Eggs, ground beef (12 percent fat or less), chicken, tuna (in water, not oil), steak, salmon, shrimp

Good carbohydrate choices: Brown rice, oatmeal, potatoes, whole wheat bread, beans

Good fat choices: Olive oil, salmon, nuts, natural peanut butter, almond butter

Incorporate the following foods into your diet to reap their many benefits:

Oatmeal/steel cut oats: Slow-burning carbohydrate for sustained energy.

Eggs: High in protein, no carbohydrates.

Nuts: Quality fats, no carbohydrates, provides a small amount of protein.

Whole wheat bagels; Slow-burning carbohydrate for sustained energy.

Lean meat/chicken: High in protein that includes many important amino acids.

Fish: High protein with healthy Omega-3 fats.

Fruits and vegetables: Nutrient dense with high-quality mineral compositions and no added sugars or chemicals.

Cottage cheese: Low-carb, high-protein snack.

Yogurt: Great source of protein, vitamins, and calcium.

Again, with each meal you're loading up on quality proteins and healthy fats while making your carbohydrate choices from the lower end of the Glycemic Index, which is an important concept to understand, and one covered later in this chapter. This provides a complete variety of nutrients and sustained energy.

Understanding Food: Protein, Fats, Carbohydrates

In the past few decades, all of the major components of the food we eat—protein, fats, and carbohydrates—have been fingered as the primary reason people are getting so fat. And oddly enough, over the past few decades, each of these same foods has also been idolized as the base for a diet that's supposedly a "sure thing" when it comes to getting healthy. In reality, protein, fats, and carbs all have a place in a healthy nutrition program. You simply need to understand each component, what it does, when it's needed, and from which sources to get it.

Carbohydrates

Carbohydrates are a wonderful source of energy for the human body, but they have been demonized more than any other part of our food supply. While the components that make up certain carbohydrate sources are bad for us, carbs in general are simply misunderstood.

When the Atkins Diet came out, people began to view carbohydrates as an evil nutrient that had to be exorcised from our diets immediately, lest we all be cursed with massive supplies of body fat that we'd be stuck with for the rest of our lives. Upon further inspection, though, things weren't so cut-and-dried. While it changed over the years, in the initial stages of the Atkins Diet, everything between the top and bottom of a McDonald's Double Quarter Pounder with Cheese was consider okay, but the bun was banned because it has carbs. And because apples and many other fruits are rich in carbs, they were considered bad, too. Something wasn't right and, fortunately, over time, people have come to a better understanding about carbohydrates.

Like any type of food, carbohydrates can be consumed in too great a quantity. Any time you consume more calories than you burn, you're going to gain weight. That's the easy part. Carbohydrates are a little more complicated because of their effect on blood sugar levels.

To see how various foods affect blood sugar levels, we use a measure called the Glycemix Index, which effectively breaks carbs into two categories: simple and complex. The Glycemic Index (GI) is a measure of how much, and how fast, a food raises blood sugar levels. It ranges between 0 and 100, with 100 being pure glucose. Pure glucose is the benchmark for the Index because it is the form of sugar our body converts carbohydrates into to burn as fuel.

Simple carbs are the kind found in candy and other junk food. They are high-GI foods, meaning they can make you feel energetic and full for a relatively short length of time, but they can greatly spike your blood sugar and can promote fat storage later on.

Complex carbohydrates, on the other hand, are low-GI foods, meaning that they are under 55 on the index. They are slow burning and provide you with lasting energy without a massive spike in your insulin levels, keeping your blood sugar at a steady flow. These types of carbs are what you'll find on the lower end of the Glycemic Index, which is where you, as a mindful, healthy eater, want to stay.

The following chart includes examples of the GI rating of various foods. When you see a reference to low-GI food or high-GI food, you'll now know what it means.

Glycemic Index Ratings: Sample High and Low Foods

Food	GI Rating
Broccoli	10
Peanuts	13
Skim Milk	27

Glycemic Index Ratings: Sample High and Low Foods

Apple, raw	40
Strawberries	40
Whole Wheat Bread	49
Brown Rice	50
Oat Bran	50
Oatmeal	51
Banana	59
Sweet corn	62
Pineapple, raw	66
White Bread	71
Watermelon	80
Rice Crispies	82
White Rice	85

Although there is a place in our diets for carbohydrates that are higher on the GI scale, the vast majority of the carbs we consume should be from the lower end of the scale.

According to GlycemicIndex.com, a low-GI diet offers the following benefits:

- Helps people lose and manage weight
- Increases the body's sensitivity to insulin
- Improves diabetes management
- Reduces the risk of heart disease
- Improves blood cholesterol levels
- Reduces hunger and keeps you fuller for longer
- Prolongs physical endurance

Protein

Proteins are made up of amino acids, which facilitate a whole host of processes in the body that revolve around muscle and tissue repair and growth. Eating chicken, fish, poultry, beef, eggs, and soy are just some of the ways you can keep a high protein intake. And a high-protein diet has been linked to more successful, longer-lasting weight loss.

There are two types of amino acids: essential and nonessential. Non-essential amino acids are those the body can synthesize itself. Essential amino acids are those we must consume through our diets. Whether an amino acid is called "essential" or not is actually a bit of a misnomer, because they are all components of good health. Amino acids play a role in healthy cellular and nervous system function, muscle and organ structure, and hormone regulation. Because of this, it's very important to get a varied mix of proteins in your diet.

Just as the hysteria surrounding carbohydrates changed the way millions of people around the world ate for many years, there has been a misconception about the consumption of protein. An unfortunate but common belief is that protein is hard on the liver, but there have been very few documented risks of consuming a high-protein diet when done so by healthy adults. The only problems have been noted when an individual has pre-existing conditions, and protein then is only one of many things that can aggravate the malady. If you have genetic predisposition to particular diseases, or if you're unsure, check with your doctor before making any dietary changes.

A vast benefit of protein is that protein-rich foods make you feel fuller, longer. Protein isn't just a bodybuilder's food; it helps create and repair muscle tissue no matter what your physique goals are, and it can help reduce body fat by controlling cravings. A great example is this: An average chicken breast has about 150 calories and about 30 grams of protein. A Coca-Cola has 140 calories and 40 grams of carbohydrates. A small, 2-tablespoon serving of peanut butter has, on average, 200 calories and 15 grams of fat. Which is going to make you more satisfied for the longest amount of time? Most people would say the high-protein chicken breast.

As discussed, key components of the gym-free and ripped program are training hard and eating right. When you train hard, you need the nutrients in your body to build muscle tissue. Protein is there for you. The next piece is eating right, ignoring cravings, and consuming proper calories. Protein, again, is a valuable part of this equation.

Fats

"Fat makes you fat," was the mantra of many health advocates for several years. As a result, dietary fat has gotten a bad rap.

Fat is a necessary component of a healthy diet. It has also been linked to improving heart health. The key is to eat the right *kinds* of fats. In doing so, you'll not only be helping your heart but also ridding your body of unwanted body fat.

Just as with carbs, not all fats are equal. You should minimize the amount of saturated fats you consume (such as coconut oil, palm kernel oil, bacon, fatty beef, cheese, and butter) and you should never eat trans fats ("hydrogenated" oils). But unsaturated fats—such as those in almonds, avocados, and olives—can be quite beneficial to the body. Of the unsaturated variety, there are monounsaturated fats and polyunsaturated fats. When you eat these types of fats, you can actually reduce your risk of heart disease by improving your cholesterol levels.

Nuts, olive oil, and many types of fish—which provide heart-healthy omega-3 fats—are all great sources of good fats. They are heart-healthy and tasty options that can improve your overall well-being and aid in restructuring your physique. (Keep in mind that farm-raised fish don't necessarily have the same omega-3 profiles that fish from the wild do. This is largely due to the huge change from their natural diets. In farm-raised varieties, fish are fed diets high in cornmeal, which creates significant change in their own nutritional composition. While you don't have to kick all farmed fish out of your diet, if meals of all wild varieties aren't feasible, do try to stick with it as much as possible.)

Water: Pure and Simple

Everyone knows you need to drink plenty of water. That doesn't mean we always do it, but even the people newest to training know they are *supposed* to. And it's true: you don't want to underestimate the role water plays in a healthy body. Staying properly hydrated has wide-ranging and significant benefits.

Water is a tool for getting fit. Not only does it quench your thirst, but it has a myriad of other benefits. A few of the most important are as follows:

- **Metabolism and hunger:** Staying hydrated helps your body maintain a normal metabolism and regulate your hunger. In other words, water helps you burn more calories and eat less.

- **Energy:** Dehydration, even to a small degree, can significantly decrease your work output and significantly *increase* the feeling of fatigue.

- **Digestion:** Water helps aid in the digestion process, which allows your body to uptake nutrients more effectively. If you're not properly hydrated, your body may not be getting all of the nutrition it needs despite your best efforts to consume the right foods.

- **Focus:** Dehydration, even to a subtle degree, has been linked to a lack of concentration and focus. If you can't put forth your best efforts in your workouts and in life in general, you're cheating yourself.

As if you needed more reasons to drink more water, in no particular order here are a couple more: it reduces the risk of certain cancers, helps detoxify the body, improves your complexion, significantly reduces joint pain, and improves circulation.

Start with eight 8-ounce glasses a day. Increase that amount to match your activity level. It really is that simple. If you haven't been drinking enough water, start now and you will be amazed at the immediate results.

Reading Food Labels

Understanding food labels is essential to building a proper diet plan. Just because something looks like it's healthy, or the package screams out "WHOLE WHEAT" in big, bold letters, doesn't mean you should eat it. Before putting any packaged food in your mouth, take a look at that black-and-white nutrition label on the side or back of the package.

First, you should know that the percentages you see on a food label are based on 2,000 calories a day. This is supposedly the average, or normal, intake according to the Food and Drug Administration (FDA). In reality, 2,000 calories probably fits a relatively small number of people with taller, active men and women often needing more than that and shorter, less active men and women needing less. It's all based on *you* and *your* lifestyle. So ignore the percentages because they probably don't apply to you. If you find that your baseline diet (which will be covered shortly) is at or around 2,000 calories, you're in luck, but for most people it's irrelevant. Instead, you should pay particular attention at the start of your new program to the following pair of items on the label.

Serving Size

People frequently overlook the recommended serving size on packaged foods. It's not uncommon for people to grab a package of something, quickly flip to the label, and see a number of calories they feel good about. The next thing you know, they've eaten the entire package. What they didn't notice was that the number of calories is based on the serving size, and that package may have contained several individual servings.

Always be sure to look at total contents as compared to serving size. For example, the label on a 20-ounce bottle of soda pop may say that it has 110 calories per serving. But that serving size is only 8 ounces. So if you drink the whole bottle, you're consuming more than twice the number of calories—and sugar—listed on the label. You may find the serving size makes that particular food not worth eating when you think of how hungry you'll still be after maxing out your desired calorie consumption.

Ingredients

Ingredients are listed in the order by which they most prominently appear in the food. So when you see sugar listed first, it means that there's a lot of it (compared to the rest of the ingredients). If you see sugar (or any of its aliases, including high fructose corn syrup) listed as the first—or often even the second—ingredient, put the package back on the shelf.

If you see the following items listed on the ingredients label, think twice before buying that product.

Hydrogenated (or partially hydrogenated) oils: Saving the long-winded, scientific explanation for academic resources, the simple explanation is that when you see the words "hydrogenated" or "partially hydrogenated" you're looking at trans fat. Avoid it. It is so bad for your health that it is highly regulated in many parts of the world.

High fructose corn syrup (HFCS): The body has little use for this simple sugar other than using it to promote fat storage. It's so common it can hardly be avoided entirely, but reducing consumption as much as possible is wise, as it is with any sugar. Steer clear wherever possible. If you want to apply one simple rule to sugar, look at it this way: less is best.

Monosodium glutamate (MSG): This ingredient is used to enhance flavor. Many people are sensitive to MSG and it can cause headaches and other maladies. Likewise, some studies suggest it has negative effects on brain cells. More studies are needed to find conclusive evidence that MSG is in fact deleterious to human health, but it's better to be safe than sorry.

This list is by no means conclusive, but following these guidelines will help you make healthier choices at the grocery store.

Label Claims

As crazy as it seems, manufacturers are allowed to put claims on their labels and packaging even if those statements aren't exactly true. The government gives food companies some leeway when it comes to their advertisements. Here's the truth behind the flashy claims:

- "Low fat" really means it has 3 grams of fat or less per serving.

- "Fat free" really means it has less than ½ gram of fat per serving.

- "Sugar free" really means it has less than ½ gram of sugar per serving.

- "Calorie free" really means it has fewer than 5 calories per serving.

- "Cholesterol free" really means it has less than 2 milligrams of cholesterol per serving.

Clearing Up Popular Food Myths

Everyone has their favorite food fact they try to live by and share with their friends whenever possible. Unfortunately, some of these "facts" are more mythical than anything else and should be dispelled. I've included a few of my favorites here:

All alcohol is detrimental to your health. In general, the calories that come from drinking alcohol are relatively empty and not exactly going to contribute to developing your ideal physique. But that doesn't mean the occasional adult beverage is going to derail your progress if you're a healthy adult.

Red wine is a great example of an alcoholic drink that actually has value. It's high in antioxidants, which have been shown time and time again to be heart-healthy. So while it's not advisable to slam down drinks like a wild college kid, a beer or glass of wine here or there is most definitely okay.

Food color means a lot. The colors of our foods have always had a weird place in the perception of nutrition, and food companies know this. If it's a vegetable and it's green, it's perceived to be healthy. If it looks like water and it's clear, we assume it's okay to drink. If it's a brown carbohydrate source, we conclude it's healthy. But in doing so, we would be wrong.

All brown products are made with whole grains. People love the term "whole grain." They know they're supposed to eat whole grains, and they see "whole grain" as being brown. Unfortunately, the companies trying to sell you their products know this and take advantage of it. That's why they might add a touch of brown food coloring to a loaf of white bread. Check the labels to ensure that "Whole Grain" is actually included, because a lot of foods that *look* healthy are made from nothing more than aesthetically improved white flour.

Brown sugar is better than white sugar. This is another color myth. People often assume that brown sugar is somehow nutritionally superior to white sugar. By and large, that's incorrect. Brown sugar is essentially a simple combination of white sugar and molasses. And while molasses has a small amount of minerals in it, it certainly doesn't add enough to boost sugar into the "healthy" category of anyone's chart.

Brown eggs are better than white eggs. A common myth is that if it costs more, it's better for you. And brown eggs almost always cost more than regular white eggs in the supermarket, so surely that logic extends to eggs, right? Wrong. Shell coloring has no bearing on the nutritional value of an egg. The color of an egg's shell only tells you the breed of hen it came from—nothing more, nothing less.

Too much protein is bad for your body. Okay, we've all heard it: protein is hard on the body. Kidneys, liver, whatever organ someone wants to choose as they tell the story, protein has somehow ruined the life of a guy who was a friend of a friend … you get the idea. But for the healthy individual, it's all nonsense.

No reliable, peer-reviewed studies have shown realistic amounts of protein intake—as high as a gram per pound of body weight—to be detrimental to health in adults with normal kidney function. High protein intake has been shown to affect kidney function for people who already had impairments with kidney function, but even then protein was only one of many things that were shown to aggravate their conditions.

The simple truth is that in normal, healthy adults, moderate to high protein intake from a variety of quality sources—not just red meat—is great for your health and your physique.

Liquid diets are successful. Liquid diets, celebrity diets—call them whatever you want—they have been all over infomercials for the last decade. They promise losing as much as 10 pounds (or more) in as little as a week. Wow, what a deal, right? But what these ads aren't telling you is that liquid diets are often packed with ingredients designed to cleanse the intestines of water and waste. You might end up with a smaller number on the scale, but only as a result of waste and water reduction. It's not body fat you lost, it's hydration, and that's not a good thing. Remember, if it sounds too good to be true, it probably is.

Nuts are fattening. Nuts contain fat, so many people shun them to avoid gaining weight. But if you listen to that balderdash, you're missing out on a great source of *healthy* fats that have been shown to do things like improve your lipid profile.

The only problem with eating almonds, peanuts, walnuts, or any other nut of choice is that it's easy to eat too many of them because they taste so good. And by volume they do pack a lot of calories, so you can easily take in too many if you don't pay attention. And that's where the weight gain can come from: excess calories. But this doesn't just apply to nuts. If you eat too many calories of *any* kind of food, whether it be eggs, chicken, fruit, or nuts, you'll gain weight. Just don't blame one particular food for it.

Eat This, Not That

We've covered a lot of information on nutrition already, but another simple tip for rapidly changing your body composition is simply to substitute foods of lower quality for better foods. This is a quick and easy change that pays dividends in the long run by removing unnecessary sugars, chemicals, and calories from your diet. Here are some simple substitutions:

Instead of:	Use:
Processed peanut butter	Natural/organic peanut butter
Soda	Sugar-free iced tea
Candy	Peanuts
Cheese	Fat-free cheese
Regular salad dressing	Fat-free dressing
White rice	Brown rice
White bread	Whole grain bread
Sugary packaged cereal	Oatmeal or homemade granola

Protein Supplements

Over the years the health food industry has introduced a wide variety of on-the-go meal options as well as post-workout recovery snacks. These have come in the form of liquids, bars, capsules, and tablets. The most effective, as well as the most studied, are protein supplements. These can serve as a great meal when you need one as well as a fantastic option to consume immediately after a workout to kick-start muscle recovery and growth.

Because protein supplements are so popular, there has been some mis-information that has made its way into popular culture that needs to be confronted so you have the most up-to-date and quality information.

There has been a presumption in the past that protein is protein, pure and simple. If it says 40g of protein, then it's 40g of protein; it doesn't matter if it's whey protein concentrate, whey protein isolate, casein protein, egg albumin, or even soy protein (the five most popular varieties of protein).

Here's the simple fact: they are *not* the same.

For the discerning trainer, I provide the following simple list.

Whey protein isolate: Whey isolate is the fastest-acting protein you can find as well as the most anabolic protein supplement source available. It is perfect for immediate consumption post-workout to help recover and deliver vital amino acids to your body.

Whey protein concentrate: Whey concentrate is also whey protein, but because whey is a by-product of milk, there are different amounts of lactose and fat in its variations. Concentrate simply has more lactose and fat than isolate. Isolate may contain 90 to 95 percent pure protein, while concentrate may be as low as around 75 percent depending on the brand.

Casein protein: Casein is the main protein found in milk. Because of the way it reacts in the body, it digests slowly compared to whey protein. As such, this type of protein is employed in situations where a training athlete is unable to consume an adequate meal for an extended period, such as prior to bedtime. Casein is highly anti-catabolic and can keep amino acid levels in the body high for as many as seven hours post-consumption. Consuming this before sleep will help feed your muscles through the night.

Soy protein: Easily the best non-animal protein source, soy is another option on the market. While it does lack a complete amino acid profile, it employs a strong antioxidant profile that can have a variety of benefits in the body. This protein also has been shown to digest nearly as well as other proteins, though it can have estrogenic effects. That said, for vegetarian and vegan trainers, this is a quality go-to protein.

Fighting Cravings

By this point, you have a great grasp of the role of nutrition for losing body fat and gaining muscle. But all the knowledge in the world can't do the work for you. And the road won't always be smooth.

The biggest obstacle to getting the body you want isn't the training. Training is fun. People who think exercise is a pain aren't doing it right. Exercise releases endorphins that make the body and mind feel *good*. That's why people who take the initiative to start training regularly stick with it—because they want that feeling again and again. It's a natural high. Once you start and get serious, training becomes as natural as breathing.

The part that's tough for anyone is fending off those nasty little cravings that sneak up without warning. You might be feeling great, have stuck with your nutrition program all day, have drunk plenty of water like you know you should, and even had a great training session earlier in the day. And then suddenly you walk in the door and your spouse surprises you with a fresh batch of cookies or an ice-cold beer. You were not even thinking about cookies or beer five minutes prior, but now that they're in front of you, you're suddenly craving them. What do you do? Simply put, man up and turn them down. Use your mental strength to stick with your plan. Consistent healthy behavior is what adds up to those awesome results. Don't let a craving ruin it.

Sometimes you just have to get upset with yourself and put your own proverbial foot down. First, try to avoid these situations whenever possible. Let your spouse or partner know that you're cleaning up your diet and it's helpful to just not have those things in the house. Or, if they're happy eating them, ask them to not tempt you by offering you some. If that doesn't work, or you find yourself away from home and often tempted, ask yourself the following simple questions:

> "What good comes from eating this? What lasting satisfaction do I get from it?"

You know that having the body of your dreams is something you get a lot of joy out of. There's nothing narcissistic about it; you earned it, so be proud of it. There's a great sense of satisfaction and happiness that comes from what you've crafted your body into. Does eating the food that is tempting you help you achieve the body of your dreams? Will you even remember what the beer or cookies tasted like in 10 minutes? No, of course not, and if you think so, take it a step further.

How many foods can you actually describe the taste of? Those are the foods you really like. The rest are merely foods you're conditioned to eat. That may sound weird, but break it down. Cake, for example, can mean hundreds of different things, but most people think about it and say, "Yeah, I like cake." So naturally if you're around it, you think, "I really like cake, I really want to eat that."

But do you actually like the specific kind in front of you, or do you just like cake in general?

Everyone who has ever been on a diet knows what this situation is like. You know you like cake or, for another example, cookies. But cake and cookies aren't individual food items; you might absolutely love chocolate chip cookies, but not care much for oatmeal cookies. That doesn't necessarily stop you from wanting to eat oatmeal cookies if someone offers you some. You might think, "Well, I do like cookies, I'll just have a couple." Once you realize the specific thing that is tempting you isn't really all that special to you, the craving will pass quickly. In instances where you're next to something that you really do enjoy, just distance yourself from it. For example, if you're at a party, simply remove yourself from the kitchen when you carry on your conversation.

There are also some things you can do to help yourself fight off cravings that extend beyond the mental aspect. Here are three easy ones you can try today:

Drink water. Studies have shown that people who drink two cups of water before each meal eat as much as 40 percent fewer calories throughout the day than others who don't drink water prior to eating. And despite the reduction in calories, people who do this generally report the same feeling of satiety as those who consume more solid foods.

Chew gum. This one may sound simple, but many people who are currently overweight are simply in the habit of constantly putting flavored foods in their mouths. While chewing gum you get flavor, which your body is after, and it keeps you busy while remaining near calorie-free.

Take a nap. A lack of sleep—which is a problem most adults face—is directly related to overeating. One way the body responds to a lack of energy is to eat, so if you're not well rested, you're going to have cravings. Additionally, it's simple timing; the longer you're up, the more likely you are to graze in the kitchen. If you have the opportunity to nap during the day, even if it's just during the weekends, take advantage of it. Your body—and your waistline—will thank you.

This book certainly isn't a text on psychology, but if you have ever tried to diet before, then you know it can be hard to stick with. The challenge is in your mind, so it's just as beneficial to train mentally as it is physically. Knowing what you'll come up against and how to handle it is an important aspect of training.

Metabolism Tricks: Speed Up Yours, Fast!

With proper nutrition you're well on your way to your ideal physique. However, there's nothing wrong with doing a few things along the way to give yourself a little extra edge. Here's a list of a few foods you can consume and things you can do to pep up your metabolism. None of these actions are going to slice the fat off in droves right away, but over time it all adds up. Remember: fitness is a marathon, not a race!

Add spice. Hot and spicy foods have been shown to increase your body's core thermal temperature, which, in turn, actually helps to burn body fat by increasing the amount of energy the body uses. For example, capsaicin, which is the pungent component of red pepper, has been shown to suppress appetite and increase satiety during a negative calorie balance.

Drink green tea. Like capsaicin, green tea has been shown to increase metabolism as well as help blunt the body's hunger response.

Get plenty of sleep. Inadequate rest will slow your metabolism down significantly, causing a lack of energy as we've already discussed. Ensure that you're getting proper rest and recovery time, not just from training but from all of life's stresses. If you're getting less than six hours of sleep per night, you're at a much higher risk of suffering some negative effects not just on your metabolism, but also your mental focus and energy levels.

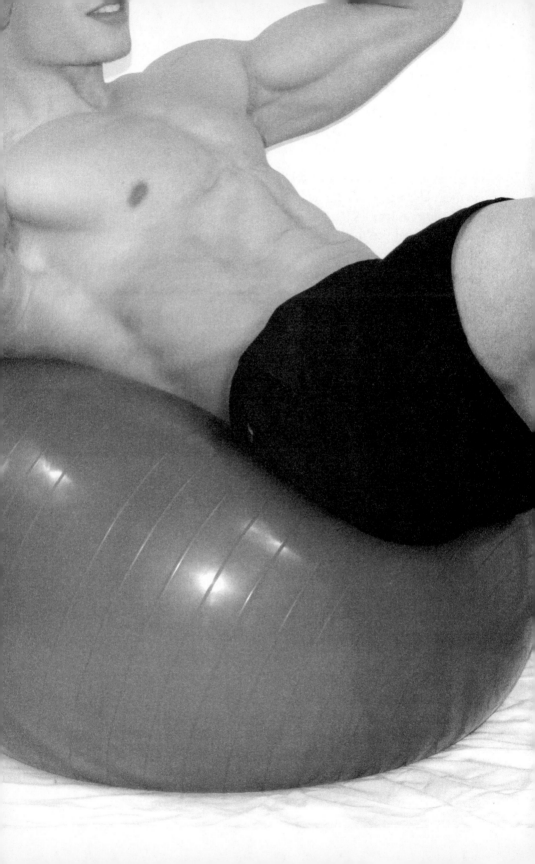

3

Getting Moving, Growing Stronger

Not everyone wants to look like a bodybuilder, but that doesn't mean you shouldn't build some quality muscle. That's because to reach your desired body type, you probably have to shed body fat. And adding muscle is one of the best ways to lose fat. Not only does more lean body mass (muscle) cause your body to burn more calories throughout the day, but high-intensity training, such as weight training, causes a lasting elevation in energy expenditure.

Excess Post-exercise Oxygen Consumption

You don't want to burn calories only while you're training. You will never get the results you're after if the only effective part of your training is while you're in motion. The real trick to achieving your goals is to ensure that what you do while you're training also pays off *after* your training is over. This comes down to something called Excess Post Oxygen Consumption, usually referred to by its initials: EPOC.

In short, EPOC is work your body does even after you're done working out. That's because the body has to repair itself and restore spent fuel, which causes a much higher rate of oxygen processing. This uses more energy, and thus burns more calories. Some studies have shown that thanks to EPOC, metabolism can be increased by nearly 15 percent for hours after training. So with that knowledge in mind, let's get to the real work!

Warm-Up: The Standard Seven

Many people think that stretching is a way to get prepared for exercise, but that's not the case. In fact, stretching without a prior warm-up puts you at serious risk for injuries. An active warm-up is actually the best way to prevent injury from exercise. A proper active warm-up consists of light movements for your entire body, even if you're only training a specific muscle group. These movements keep you in motion—hence the term *active*—and prepare all of your interconnected muscles for training. This enables your blood to flow and your entire body to work together more freely. This is especially important because even if you're doing exercises that target a specific area, various other parts of your body are always involved in some way or another.

Stretching before doing any sort of warm-up can be risky because you immediately put stress on your muscles. Think of it as jumping out of bed in the morning and trying to train immediately; it would be extremely uncomfortable and you're much more likely to pull or strain a muscle. On the other hand, if you go about your day for a bit, go through some easier and lighter motions, then your body is prepared and your subsequent training is much easier and safer. (See Chapter 4 for a detailed discussion of stretching.)

Spend a few minutes working through the following seven-step warm-up routine before your training and/or stretching sessions. It only takes a couple of minutes and is a great way to get your muscles and joints warmed up and limber.

Step 1: Knee Lifts

Do this lower body warm-up movement either standing in place or while walking. Slowly and gently lift your knees, one at a time, up in front of you just until you feel a bit of tension in your hamstrings and glutes. Alternate legs until you have done at least 10 raises with each leg.

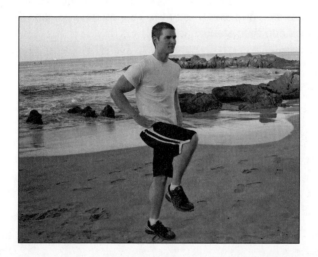

Step 2: Slow Bends

Stand with your feet shoulder-width apart and a slight bend in your knees, with your arms out in front with your palms facing your body. Slowly—try to make it last a full 3 seconds—bend at the waist so your fingertips move toward the top of your feet. When you feel your hamstrings tighten a bit, pause, then return to your starting position again with a three-count. Do 10 to 15 of these bends each warm-up session.

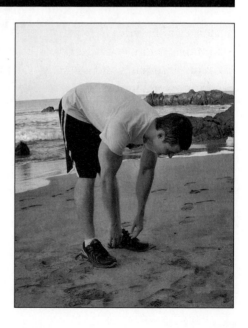

Step 3: Back Squeeze

On the last repetition of your slow bends, move right into this back and rear-deltoid warm-up movement. Remain bent at the waist with your back flat and your arms hanging in front of you. Place your palms together and then slowly pull each arm back as if you are squeezing your shoulder blades together. When you have pulled back as far as you can comfortably go, hold there for a moment, and slowly return to your starting position. Repeat this 10 to 15 times and then stand.

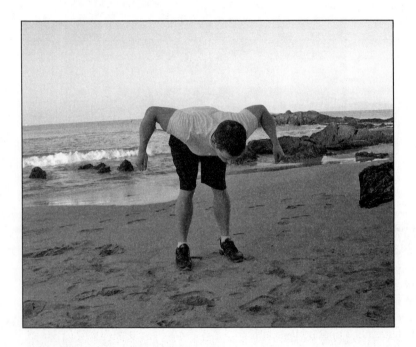

Step 4: Five-Tier Squat

To help ensure the safety of your knees when training, you'll want to slowly work them through a full range of motion. To do so, slowly bend at the knees while keeping your hands on your hips and your back straight. Only squat slightly on your first bend, then return to your starting position. Squat a bit lower on the second repetition, then a little more on the third, slightly more on the fourth, and the fifth should have you squatting to a "seated" position. After the fifth squat, start over with the first tier once more and repeat in descending fashion. Work through at least four five-tier squats to properly warm up.

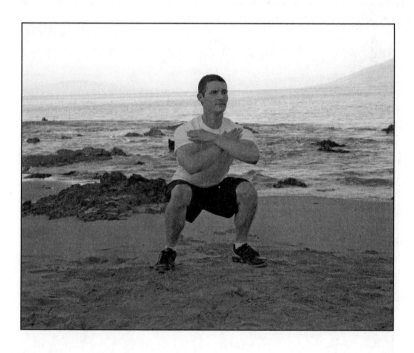

Step 5: Shoulder Claps

To give your shoulders a good warm-up, start with your arms out to your side and bent up at the elbows (like an "L" shape). With your hands open flat and your palms facing forward, slowly raise your arms while rotating your hands to face each other until they meet and "clap" directly above your head, and then return to the position in which you began. Do this for 10 repeats.

(This is a variant of the shoulder press movement with dumbbell weights discussed later in this book, but in that exercise don't touch the weights together as the extra weight of the dumbbells will stress the shoulders and rotator cuffs.)

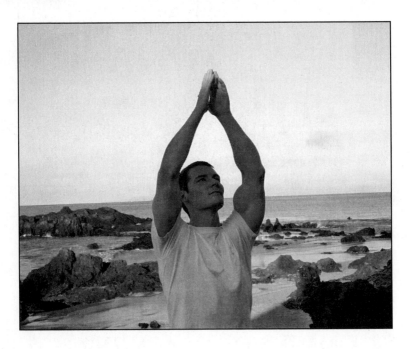

Step 6: Straight-Arm Circles

Place your arms straight out in front of you, palms facing down, and move your arms in small circles for up to 10 seconds at a time.

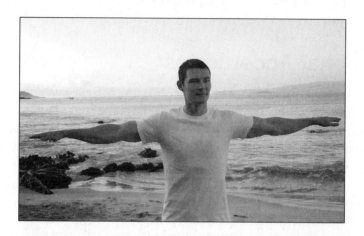

Step 7: Five-Tier Presses

The final warm-up exercise is a variation of the push-up. Move to your knees—even if you're perfectly capable of standard push-up presses—and place your hands on the ground in the push-up position. Just like the five-tier squat, you're going to lower yourself to five different levels. The first will be just a small, gentle bend, and each subsequent press will lower you slightly more. By the fifth press, you should pause with your chest only a couple of inches from the ground.

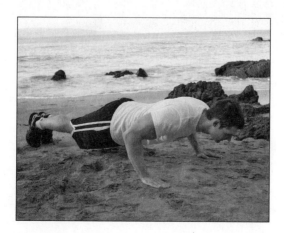

After you have completed these seven warm-ups, stand up, move around, and see how your body feels. If you feel warm and loose, let the training begin. If you still feel a bit tight, rest for a minute and repeat the warm-ups until you're ready to move into the workout.

Optional Accessories

Training at home doesn't mean you can't use some gym-quality equipment. The aim of this book is to show you how easy and fun it is to get in shape from your own home or even hotel rooms while you're traveling. That said, some people enjoy adding a few tools to their training regimen while others like to stick with the traditional body weight routines. As long as you train hard and consistently, you'll get in—and stay in—fantastic shape.

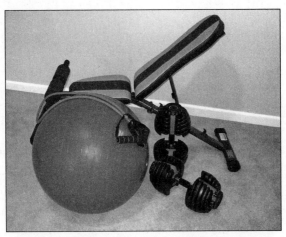

A fitness ball, stretch cord, adjustable dumbbells, and a workout bench are all optional accessories you can use to enhance your workout.

Adjustable Dumbbells

When adjustable dumbbells were introduced years ago they were big, bulky, and expensive. Although you had a variety of weights you could use for a multitude of exercises at home, you never really were able to get that "in the gym" experience because the equipment just wasn't very functional. Fortunately, exercise technology has caught up with demand, and today it's possible to find a number of quality, affordable adjustable dumbbell sets on the market. For the price of just a few months' gym membership you can bring the gym right to you.

If you don't understand an exercise, re-read the material and study the accompanying illustrations before attempting the movement. None of these exercises should feel awkward or painful, so stop immediately if you experience any severe discomfort.

BOSU and Fitness Balls

Though it's called a "ball," a BOSU ball is really only half of a ball resting on a flat, sturdy platform. The upper half, which is round, rubber, and malleable, requires users to activate a variety of muscles to stabilize themselves. You can also flip the BOSU upside down, placing the flat side upward, and perform a variety of exercises on the ball that way.

A fitness ball, also sometimes called a "stability ball," is used for core stabilizing exercises. It's basically a giant rubber ball, with no flat surface on any side. Because it places the user higher off the ground than the BOSU, this ball is generally preferred when training the abdominals. It can also be used in place of a bench for many exercises.

Incorporating BOSU and fitness balls can be a fun way to spice up your workout, but you should not conduct all of your training with them. To get the best results from working out, you need to keep the body guessing with new and exciting ways of exercising. Since you spend the majority of your day on solid ground, you should conduct the majority of your training on solid ground. The real benefit of BOSU and fitness balls is that they target stabilizing muscles, which are generally smaller and harder to target, but they also require lower volume to sufficiently train.

Lastly, always keep in mind that an unstable surface is not a natural plane. Even after you've become well versed in balancing yourself and working out with the BOSU or fitness ball, don't overexert yourself or try anything that causes discomfort. You may have seen people doing heavy barbell squats while standing on a fitness ball, but while impressive, the risk for serious injury by doing an exercise like that far outweighs the benefits. So, as with anything, when employing new techniques, start slow and always think safety first.

Stretch Cord

One of the more useful accessories to your training is nothing more than a simple piece of stretchable rubber called a *stretch cord*. You can buy them at any store that sells fitness equipment, but you might even have something around the house that can accomplish the same tasks. One caveat: make sure it's strong enough so that you don't risk it breaking while you're using it. You can seriously injure yourself if something were to snap back at you with enough force. That said, using a stretch cord not only enhances certain exercises but enables you to do entirely new exercises.

Upper Body Exercises

Having a strong and well-developed upper body isn't just about looking good. Strengthening your shoulders, arms, chest, and back makes everyday tasks much simpler and also helps prevent injuries. Whether you're an athlete or just want to put on some lean mass, there are plenty of ways to improve your body from the waist up.

The rest of this chapter describes a wide variety of exercises you can do at home. Later on, in Chapter 6, I help you put together a workout routine using these exercises. These exercises are *not* intended to be done in the order they are described here, and you will notice in Chapter 6 the workouts are quite varied to keep your routine interesting and to keep improving your physique as you develop stronger, more ripped muscles.

Arms: Biceps, Triceps, and Forearms

Although they're the smaller of the upper body muscles, the arms—your biceps, triceps, and forearms—get the lion's share of attention when you're on the beach or just out and about. That's because they're shown off; you can surely hide an undeveloped chest or back under a t-shirt, but especially during the summertime your arms are there for all to see. This has caused a lot of people to place undue emphasis on their arms and neglect other large important muscle groups. Remember that the key to overall health and fitness is to give every muscle its fair share of attention, and not focus on certain parts. That said, quality arm training is important to your everyday lifestyle because strong arms make simple tasks easier and safer. The forearms are particularly important to grip strength—which is quite important in many occupations—and the upper arms are always getting the heavy loads when carrying or moving things. And while biceps tend to get the most attention, it's actually the triceps that make up the vast majority of arm size. This is just another reason why focusing on *all* of your muscles pays off: they all work together!

Traditional Curls

The simplest exercise for the biceps is also the most effective. Simply by way of how the muscle contracts, almost any biceps exercise you'll ever see will be similar to the traditional curl.

Stand tall or sit upright with your back flat and take an object in hand. Curl the weight upward, pausing at the peak of contraction, and lower the arm back to the starting position.

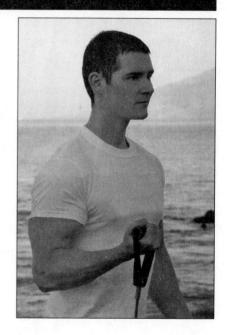

Freeman Curls

Freeman curls are a great biceps exercise using relatively low weight. They are very similar to the traditional curl, but the key is in the mechanics.

Take a weight in hand—one in each hand if you have equal weights—and sit in a straight-backed chair. Ensure you have perfect posture and place your arms at your sides. Making sure your elbows don't move at all, curl your arms up and pause at the top, lowering back down to starting position slowly. Don't lock out completely in between reps to ensure you keep constant tension on the muscle.

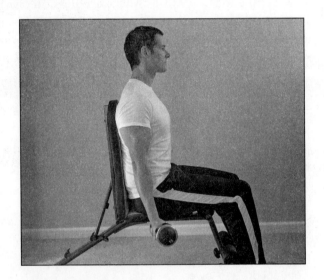

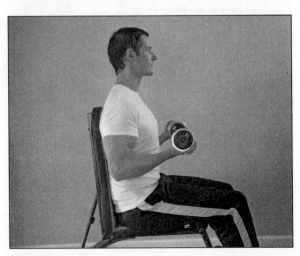

Doorknob Curls

Crouch down so that you're facing the knob-side of a door. Grab each handle with a palms-up grip and lean back so your arms are extended. Bend from the elbow down, drawing yourself toward the door. Slowly return yourself to the starting position.

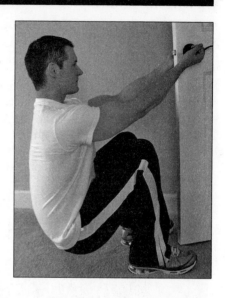

Towel Curls

From a seated position on the floor, place a towel around the underside of one foot, gripping the towel on either side with an underhand grip. Lift the leg to a "two o'clock" position and lean back until your arms are extended. Without allowing the knee to bend, curl your arms to draw your body forward. You will know you are doing this properly when you feel the burn in your arms, and not in your abs.

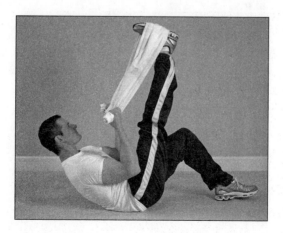

Hammer Towel Curls

This exercise can be done with a towel or even an old shirt and is particularly effective if the item of clothing is made out of a bit of nylon or polyester to allow for a little bit of give (but is also why you want to use an *old* shirt).

Hold one end of the material in one hand at your side. Cross the other arm in front of your body and grab the other end. Using the arm that is crossing your body and leaving the elbow in place, draw ("curl") the hand upward. You will be curling against resistance you create, so make it reasonably challenging. The stretching material becomes beneficial here because it takes a little of the human element out while still allowing you to control the difficulty.

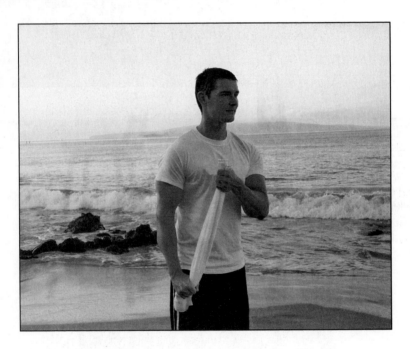

Cord Curls

Place a stretch cord or similar material on the ground and stand on the middle of the cord. Take an end of the cord in each hand, positioned so that as you curl your hands upward, the cord provides resistance.

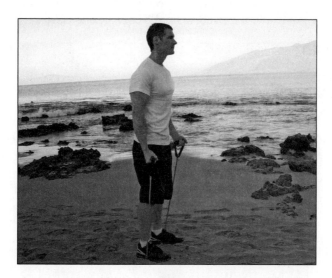

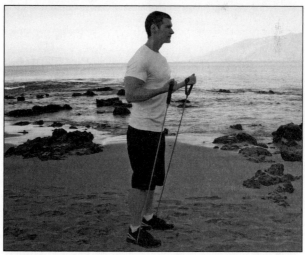

Extended Curls

Attach a stretch cord to something solid about shoulder height (alternatively you can start from your knees, so you may affix it on a shorter object). Take the cord and position yourself so that your arm is extended straight out in line with your shoulder. Keep your elbow in place and curl your arm back as if you were going into a traditional front biceps flexing pose.

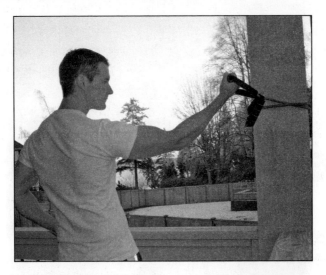

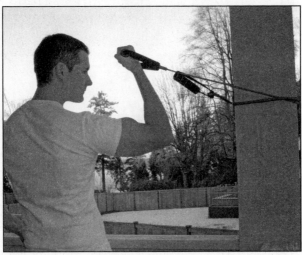

Triceps Push-up

A simple tweak on the standard push-up allows you to go from targeting the chest to working your triceps with a phenomenal exercise. Instead of placing your arms outside of your body, bring them closer together so that they extend straight down from your shoulders. From here, move your hands back until they are lined up under your pecs. Slowly lower yourself to the same height above the ground as on a standard push-up, and also maintain a slight bend in your elbow at the top of the push-up.

Tip: When doing this exercise, do not allow your elbows to flare out. Doing so will take the tension off of the triceps and also create the potential for injury.

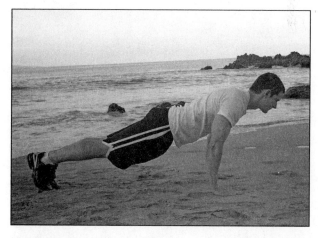

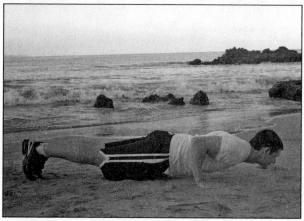

Triceps Dips

Find a relatively low platform or seat that is solidly placed. Place your palms on it so that your fingers point and fall over and down its edge. Face away from the platform and support yourself on nearly extended arms while extending your legs straight out in front of you. Lower yourself until your butt is just above the ground, pause, and return to the starting position. Ideally you will be using an object high enough that allows your triceps to become parallel with the ground when you are at the bottom of the movement.

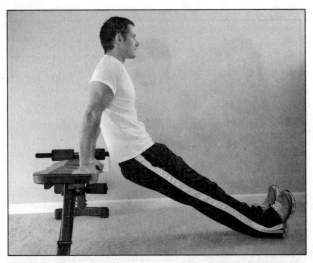

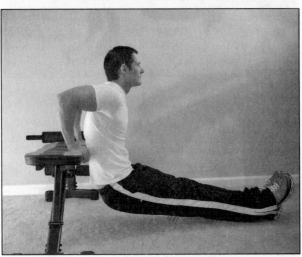

Chair Dips

In this variation on the triceps dip, place a sturdy chair on either side of you with the seat facing toward you. Grip the top of each chair's back with your hands, and extend your arms, lifting yourself up while bringing your feet up behind you. Dip down until your triceps are parallel with the floor, and return to the starting position. If you have tall chairs or barstools, you can face them so that the seat portion is on each side of you, and do the same movements with your hands on the seats.

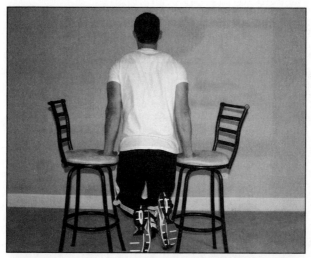

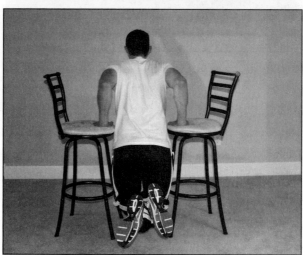

Triceps Kickbacks

For this exercise you can use a dumbbell or any object that has adequate weight and is easy to grip.

Lean forward until your back is almost parallel with the ground with one leg positioned back and your knees bent slightly to give yourself sturdy footing. Place your elbow at your side and allow the rest of your arm, with weight in hand, to hang down toward the floor. Draw your hand back with your little finger pointed upward until you feel your triceps flex. Toward the end of the movement, rotate your hand so that your palm is facing up. Slowly return to the starting position.

Alternatively, if you don't have a weighted object you may use a towel held with one end in each hand. As you draw your training arm back, use the other arm to create adequate resistance.

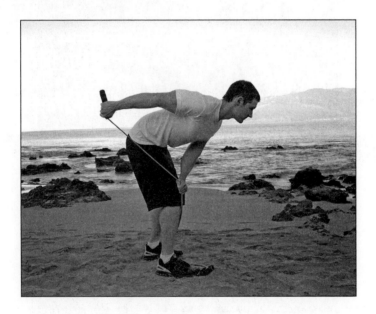

Triceps Extensions

This is best done with a couch or solid chair after you remove the cushions. Face the piece of furniture and place your hands evenly over its exposed edge. Then create a "V" shape with the rest of your body where your hips are the highest point of your body and your legs are straight. Slowly lower yourself so that your head passes down between your arms, and then press yourself back to the starting position.

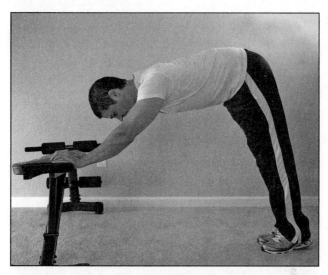

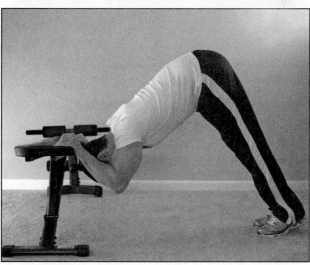

Cord Triceps Extensions

Take a cord in one hand and hold it behind your back while holding the other end of the cord straight above you with the other hand. With the extended arm, bend only from the elbow down (from elbow to your hand) behind your head, and then re-extend.

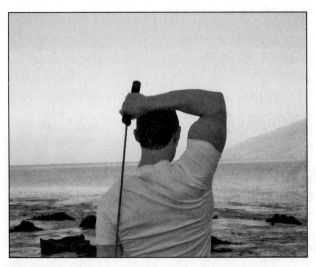

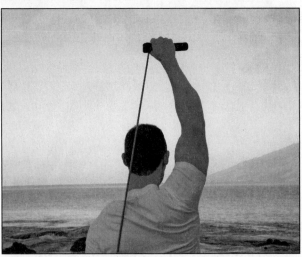

Finger Flicks

With your hands out in front of you—you can be sitting or standing—make a pair of fists. Then explode your entire hand out and extend all of your fingers and thumb completely. Then quickly make fists and "squeeze" each tightly. Repeat this exercise quickly for sets of 20 to 30 and your forearms will begin to grow with haste.

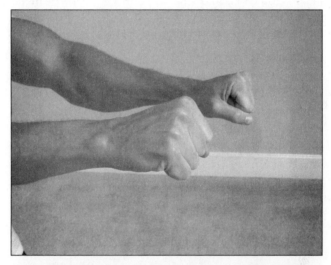

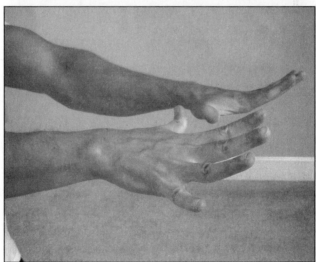

Forearm Curls

Take a weighted object that allows you to get a solid grip and hold it with your palm facing up.

Slowly curl your hand toward your body until you aren't able to draw it in any farther. Then slowly extend it back to the starting position.

Ripped addition: You can also do this by starting with the palm facing down.

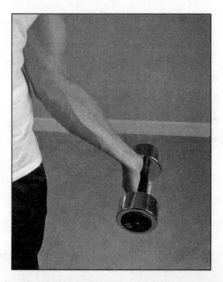

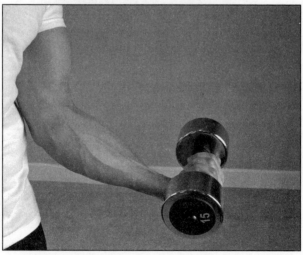

Forearm Rope Curls

This exercise may take a little craftsmanship but is easy enough to do and worth the effort. Attach a rope to a stick or short piece of piping. At the other end of the rope, attach a weight plate or other heavy object. Now, hold your arms out in front of you and roll the rope around the stick/piping, moving one hand at a time. When the object has reached the top, slowly unravel it until the item returns to the starting position. You can even attach the same duffel bag used in the standard forearm curl exercise, which offers an easy way to adjust the amount of resistance.

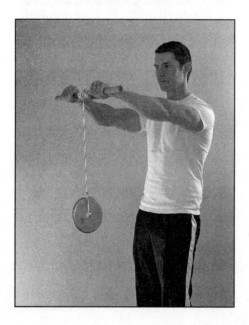

Chest

The value of a strong chest is often overlooked, but the reality is a strong set of pectorals is infinitely valuable. Whether you're pushing, pulling, or pressing, the chest comes into play. It is an extremely functional muscle group—and a well-developed chest is aesthetically impressive!

Push-up Presses

There are so many different variations of the push-up that you can almost get a complete chest workout simply by using an array of movements that all look similar. This just goes to show how a small tweak can change an entire exercise and move you to a different realm of results! Gone are the days when you needed a gym with benches and barbells; here's how to get the same results wherever you are.

The Original

Place your hands on the ground evenly outside of your shoulders and extend your body, propping yourself up on the balls of your feet. Slowly lower yourself until you're as close to the floor as possible without touching and then return to the starting position.

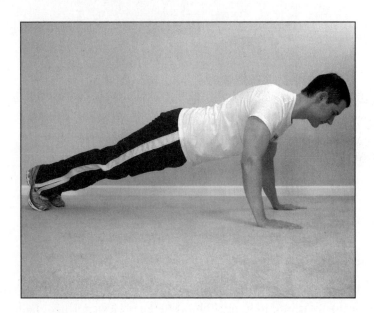

Tip: Many people make the mistake of allowing the tension to come off of the muscle when they return to the starting position by locking out the arms. Never come to a complete lockout; instead, keep your elbows slightly bent at the top of the push-up.

Ripped addition: Place your feet on an object—a couch, chair, or step—which makes your body horizontal from your head all the way to your toes. This adds leverage to your push-up and thus increases the difficulty.

The Incline

You can use any elevated platform for this variation of the push-up, which allows you to attack your chest from a new angle. You might try using a stair or perhaps a couch with the cushion removed.

This is the same as the original push-up but you are simply starting with your body on a higher plane.

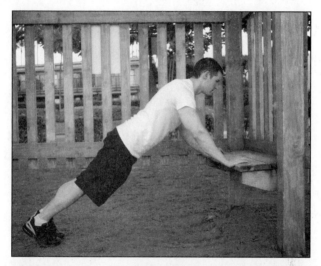

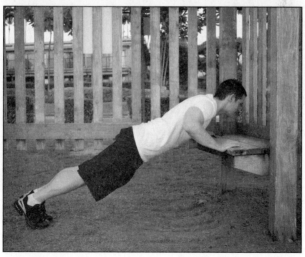

The Decline

Find an object that allows you to lift your feet 6 to 12 inches higher off the ground than your head and do push-ups from this position.

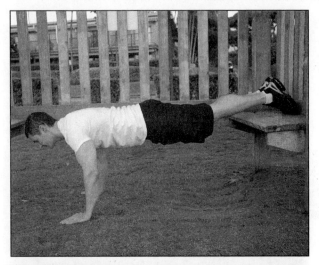

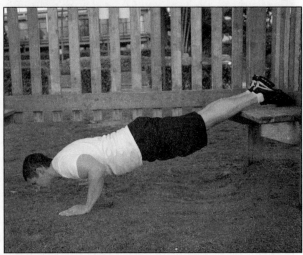

Platform Push-up

Find two objects of equal height and place them under your hands when you're doing the traditional push-up. Allow your chest to dip between the objects when lowering yourself toward the ground.

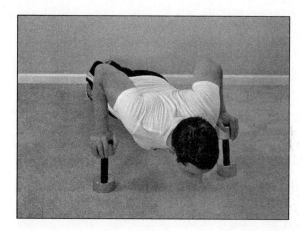

Sliding Press

Start in a traditional push-up position. Start by sliding one arm out to the side and then follow it with the upper body, bending at the elbow and doing a push-up off to that side. Return the body and arm to the original, traditional position, and alternate to the other side. This will make you feel a good bit of tension in the outer region of the pectoral muscle on the side you're bending on, and is a building exercise toward being able to do one-arm push-ups.

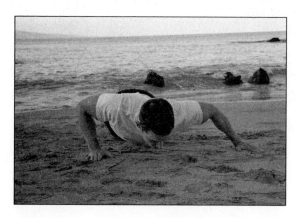

One-Arm Push-up

Position your legs a bit wider than normal to do this one-arm push-up properly. Secure the hand not being used by setting it against your lower back and push up using the other arm.

Alternatively, you can start training for this by doing it from your knees.

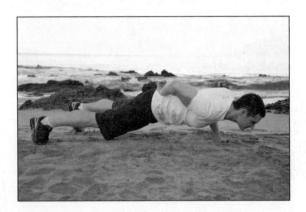

Flyes

For this particular chest exercise, you will need a smooth floor (hardwood floors are perfect). Start in the traditional push-up position but place folded-up washcloths between your palms and the floor.

Slowly allow your hands to slide out from the body until your chest is just a couple of inches off the floor, then slide your arms back to the starting position, keeping your arms slightly bent at the elbow throughout the exercise.

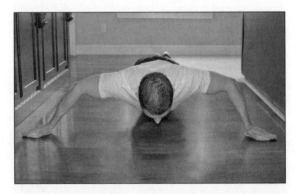

Dumbbell Fitness Ball Press

Start by sitting on a fitness ball with a dumbbell in each hand and slowly roll yourself forward with your feet until you're lying back and balancing with your feet flat on the floor, knees bent, and back flat (your upper back will be balancing on the fitness ball). Point your elbows out to your sides and line your hands and dumbbells toward the ceiling. Press the dumbbells up until your arms are nearly extended, pause, then return to your starting position.

Alternatively, you can do this with your upper body at an angle to give yourself incline press positioning.

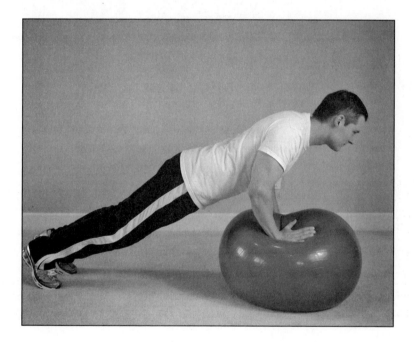

Tension Pull

This is a static exercise that can cause a great, healthy burn in your pectorals. Lie back on a solid object (an arm of a couch works, or a fitness ball or anything similar) and take the ends of a small towel into your hands. Raise your arms straight above you and pull the ends of the towel to each side. Pull for a given period of time, then press the thumb sides of your fists together and push against each other. Alternate back and forth for your set.

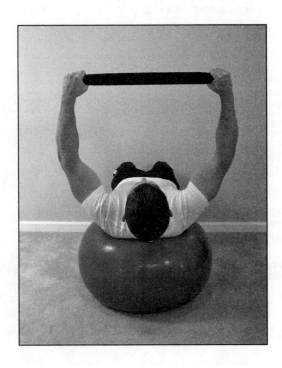

Shoulders

When looking at the shoulders, the main muscles you see are the trapezius and the deltoids. While not strictly a muscle of the shoulder, the trapezius extends from the shoulder to the neck and is functionally involved in every shoulder movement. The deltoids, which when developed are the nice, round muscles at the top of your arms, consist of three "heads," which are different sets of muscle fibers. They consist of the lateral deltoid heads (those on the sides of you), the posterior (those on the back side of the deltoid), and the anterior (those on the front side). For the most power, strength, safety, and appeal, it's important to work all three deltoid heads for complete shoulder development.

Handstand Press

You may want to place a small pillow on the floor under your head for this exercise.

Start facing a sturdy wall or closed (and locked) door. Squat down and place your hands on the ground a couple of inches away from the wall. Lean forward and put your head on the ground so that you are looking at your legs. Kick off with your legs until they touch the wall and you are upside down against the wall. Push with your arms to slowly raise and lower yourself.

In time, after you've developed balance, try doing this exercise without the aid of a wall!

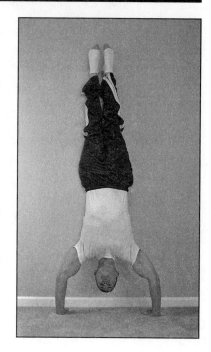

Half-Over Press

If you aren't quite ready to do handstand presses yet, this exercise will help you while still sculpting your shoulders. Find a solid object with a relatively high platform (the arm of a couch may work for you). Place your body over the edge until you are able to bend forward and place your hands on the ground while leaving your back as vertical as possible. Press your body up in the same manner as the handstand press.

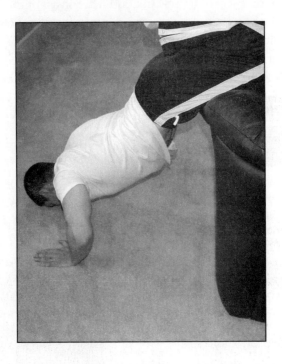

Side Lateral Raises

Take a weighted object, such as a dumbbell or other type of evenly weighted container, and hold it in one hand. Standing up tall or sitting with your back straight, raise the arm holding the object to your side. Raise your arm until your hand is slightly above your shoulder and then slowly lower it back to the starting position. Maintain a very slight bend in your elbow as you do this.

To give yourself consistent tension, don't return the weight all the way back to your side. Instead, stop just before you feel the deltoid muscle relax, and do the next repetition. Once done, repeat the exercise for the other arm.

This same exercise can be done with a stretch cord that you are either standing on one end of, or, if your cord has an attachment at one end, is affixed to your ankle.

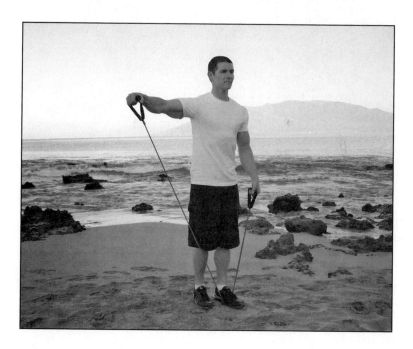

Front Lateral Raises

Take a weighted object or dumbbell in hand and stand tall. Keeping a slight bend in the elbow, raise your arm out to the front of you until your hand rises just above the level of your shoulder. Return to the starting position. Repeat for both arms.

This exercise can also be done with a stretch cord.

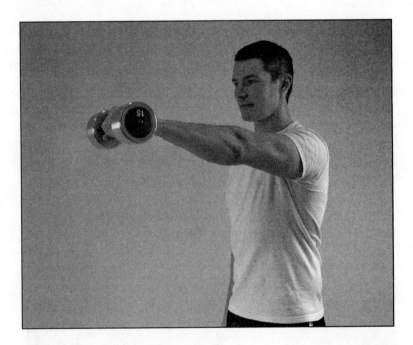

Rear Lateral Raises

You can use a stretch cord or a weighted object for this exercise.

Keeping a bend in your knees, lean forward until your back is nearly parallel with the floor. Allow the arm with the weight to hang straight down, in line with the shoulder. Draw the arm, with a slight bend in your elbow, out to the side as far as you can, pausing in the fully extended position just briefly before slowly controlling the weight back to the starting position. Repeat with the other arm.

If you are using a stretch cord, you will need to place the leg that is opposite of the working arm forward just a bit to secure the cord by standing on it. Doing so allows a straight pattern of resistance for the working muscle.

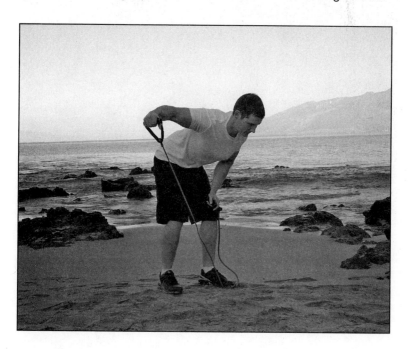

Overhead Press

From a seated position with your back flat against a chair, take two objects of equal weight into your hands. Lift your arms so that the objects nearly meet above your head, but don't allow them to touch. Slowly bring the weight down toward either side of your head, stopping when your triceps become parallel with the ground.

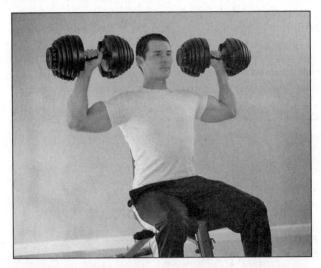

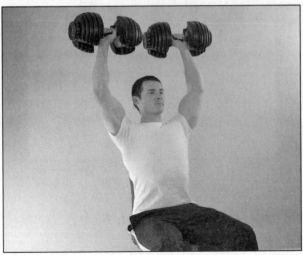

Cable Overhead Press

Place a stretch cord below you and stand on its middle. Take the ends of the cord in your hands and "raise the roof" with your hands, extending your arms upward until they are nearly straight (don't lock out your elbows).

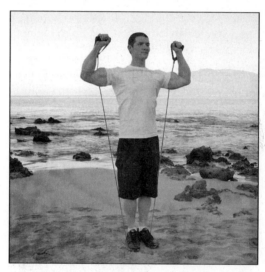

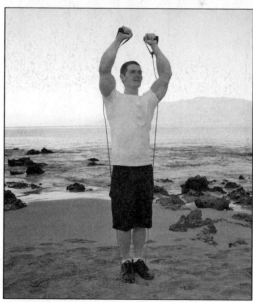

Shrugs

Shrugs can be done with equally weighted objects in each hand or with both hands sharing the weight of one object.

If you are using the two-hand method, take your weights and place them at your sides. Ensure you are standing tall with no bend in your back. Raise your shoulders as if you are trying to connect them to your ears. Do *not* roll your shoulders forward or backward.

Alternatively, if you are using one object such as a bag that has been loaded with weight, ensure your shoulders are square with your body and hold the object so that as you raise it, it comes up just barely in front of you. Ensure you aren't holding it out too far in front of you or in a position that causes you to lean. You can also do this exercise with the weights held behind your back.

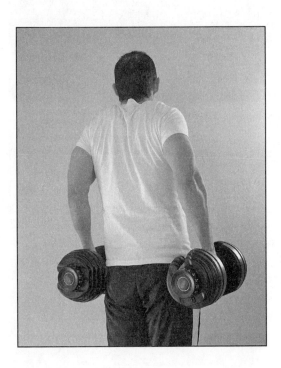

Back

Guys always get asked, "How much do you bench?" but when you're talking about stretching a t-shirt to impressive proportion, a well-developed back is what you're really looking for. The back consists of large, powerful muscles that affect everything you can do with your body. From proper posture and seated comfort to impressive musculature, working out your back is vital.

Pull-ups on Doorframes

Hang yourself from a doorframe or other elevated, stable, sturdy object. Place your arms just beyond shoulder-width and lift yourself as high as possible. Slowly lower yourself to the starting position, leaving your arms slightly bent.

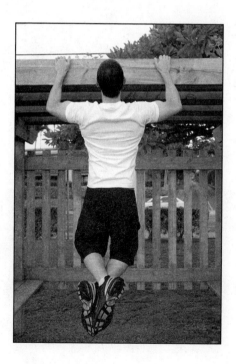

Lifted Waves

Lie on the floor facedown with your arms extended out to your sides and your palms open and flat on the ground. Lift your chest and arms as far off the ground as possible while the rest of your body maintains contact with the floor.

Keeping your arms straight and off the ground, slowly draw them back as far as possible before returning to the starting position. Do not allow your arms to touch the ground in between repetitions.

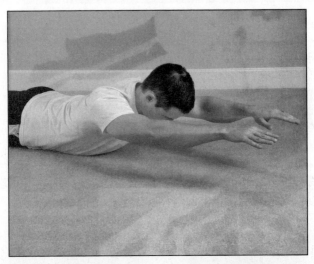

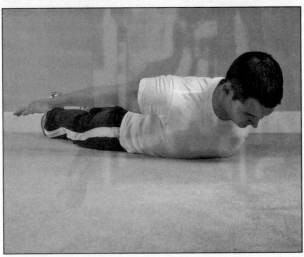

Cable Rows

Stand on the center of a cable that has been laid out on the ground. Take an end in each hand and bend forward at the waist until your upper body is at a 45-degree angle. Keeping your arms nearly straight, lift them forward as high and as evenly as possible. You will feel this exercise in your back as well as your shoulders.

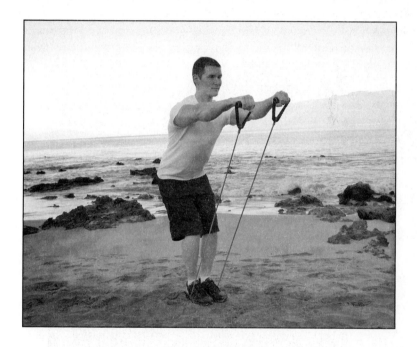

One-Arm Rows

Start by standing with your feet shoulder-width apart. Move your left foot back and out slightly until you can comfortably lean your body forward to the point where your back is close to being parallel with the floor. In this position, you should feel very sturdy.

Take a weighted object, such as a dumbbell or stuffed bag, in your left hand and allow your arm to extend straight down. Now, while gripping the weighted object, draw your arm back as if you were bringing the object into your ribs. Control the movement both in the upward and downward portions. Repeat this exercise for your right arm as well.

While conducting this exercise, your non-working-side hand can secure itself on a solid object, like a piece of furniture, or on your forward leg.

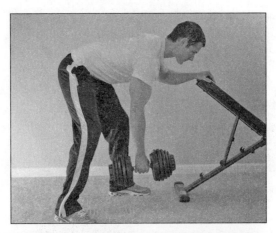

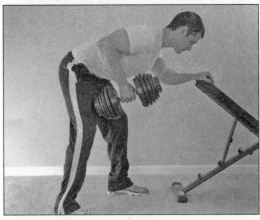

Post Rows

Depending on what's available to you, you can use a variety of different things to conduct this exercise. Anything that allows you to grip in front of you and secures your feet (such as stair railings or some pillars) will suffice. Grab a railing or post(s) in front of you (if you don't have adjoining grip options in front of you, you can place one hand above the other). Place your toes up against the object and allow your hips to drop back until both your arms and legs are extended. Pulling with your arms, bring yourself forward, focusing on using your back, not your arms, to create the motion. Your elbows should go out toward the sides rather than point toward the ground.

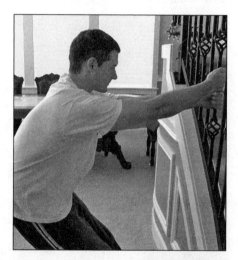

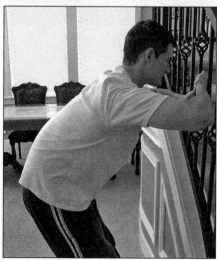

Ground Pull-ups

Set two chairs (or other equal-height objects) on either side of you while you are on the ground, flat on your back. Take a solid bar or pole and set it across the chairs. Grip the bar outside of your shoulder-width with both hands and pull yourself upward. Your body should be rigid other than your arms, and when you're in the "up" position, only your heels should be touching the ground.

Alternatively, you can do this with any two solid objects placed at your sides that you can use to reach and pull yourself up with. This can be two tables, couch or chair ends, or folding chairs (just ensure they won't fold with your weight).

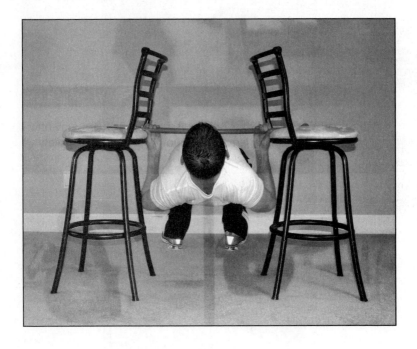

Table Pull-ups

This can be done as an alternative to the Ground Pull-ups, or, because the positioning requires an underhand grip instead of an overhand option, can be done as a separate exercise.

Lie on your back so that your chest is underneath the edge of a sturdy table (or similar object) with the rest of your body out away from the table. Reach up and grip the edge underhanded so that your fingers are on the table/surface top. Pull yourself up toward the underside of the table.

Ripped addition: Try elevating your feet.

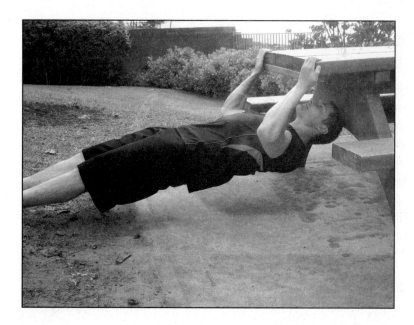

Lower Body Exercises

The legs are the driving force of your entire body. Having powerful legs makes everything else you do, from walking upstairs to carrying something heavy, easier.

Traditionally, legs have unfortunately been an afterthought by guys just wanting big chests and large arms. Those with truly impressive physiques are well balanced and have filled-out legs to match wide shoulders and arms, giving that "X-Frame" look. And you can build great legs right from home.

Quadriceps, Hamstrings, and Hips

The main components of the upper leg are your quadriceps—the muscles on the front of your thigh—and the hamstrings, which are the muscles on the back side of your thigh. It's important to develop these muscles together rather than focusing on one or the other, because they have a very synergistic relationship. Not only will you be more comfortable when giving each group proper attention, but your legs will also come to look more complete and detailed.

Squats

Easily the most basic leg exercise out there, squats have a huge number of variations you can use to attack your legs from new angles and inspire new growth. Even so, you'd be hard pressed to beat the traditional squat in effectiveness.

Start by standing with your legs just outside shoulder-width. You may keep your hands at your hips, across your chest, or even extended out in front of you, if you'd like. Keeping your feet flat on the ground, bend at the knees and lower your hips—keeping your back straight—until your hips reach about the height of the knees. Pushing from the bottom of your feet, drive yourself back to the standing position.

Ripped addition: Take dumbbells or equal weights in either hand and rest them on/against your shoulders during your squats. You can also add weight to a backpack for increased resistance, but wear the backpack on the front of your body to ensure the weight doesn't throw you off balance.

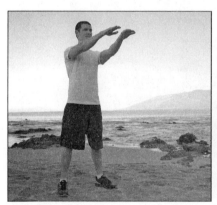 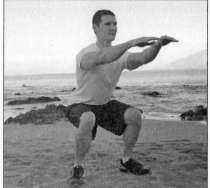

Lunges

Lunges are a classic and extremely effective leg exercise. Start by standing normally with your hands on your hips (alternatively, you can do this with weights in each hand and your arms at your side). Take a big step forward with one foot and bend at that knee, keeping the shin vertical, until the knee of your opposite leg almost touches the ground. From here, you can either step back to the starting position, or you can push off with the front leg and into the next step and repeat the technique with your opposite leg.

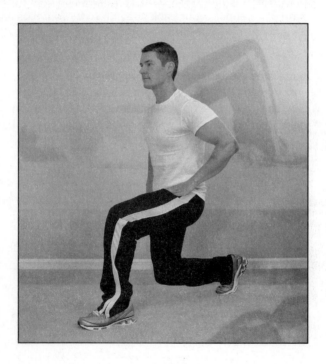

Knee Drop

This exercise is a cross between a squat and a lunge, but it targets muscles in your legs in a unique way that makes this a great addition to any leg workout, even if you're already doing squats and lunges.

Start standing up straight with your feet together. Place one leg about one foot forward and slide the other back until it's far enough that bending that knee would place it next to and just behind the rear of your forward foot. That motion is actually what you will be doing. Bend the rear leg until it hovers just above the ground, pause briefly, then using only the strength from that leg, press yourself back up to starting position. Repeat this for a complete set before switching and rotating sides.

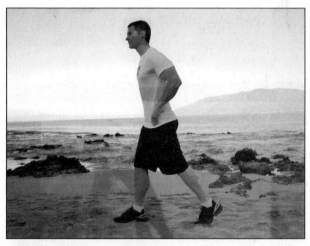

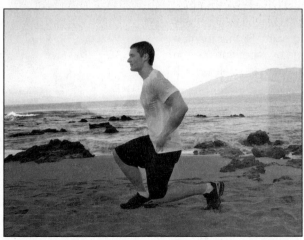

Riding Stance

This is an endurance-based exercise that will make your quads burn. Stand with your feet a few inches outside of shoulder-width and "sit" down until your quadriceps are parallel with the ground. Make sure that you keep your back straight and don't lean forward.

Ripped addition: To really test yourself, get a paper or plastic cup and set it on the top of your leg once you get into position. It will keep you honest because the cup will tip if you begin to cheat and start standing up.

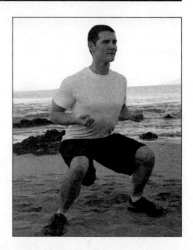

Slow Stepping

For a fantastic way to build your legs, find a set of stairs or a raised platform that is wide and sturdy. Place one foot on the platform and keep your hands on your hips. While maintaining solid footing, slowly lift yourself up until you are able to touch the toe of your free-hanging leg to the heel of the foot on the platform. Then, slowly lower yourself to your starting point. Rather than alternating legs by repetition, perform your full set of one leg before switching to the other.

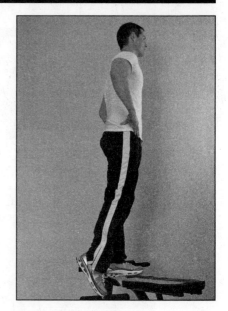

Platform Lift

Set a solid, flat object—such as a bench—at your side. Try to make the level of the object about even with your knee, although a little higher or a little lower is feasible as well.

Standing sideways to the bench, place the bottom of one foot on the center of the bench and lift yourself up. The foot not balancing on the bench should gently touch the inside of the balancing foot and then return to the ground. Return to the starting position and repeat.

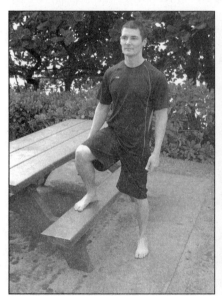 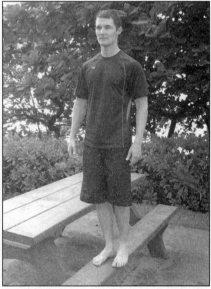

Single-Leg Straight Bend

Similar to the slow bends done in the warm-up, this exercise uses leverage to put more tension on the hamstrings, resulting in a greater workout.

Start with your legs lined up with your shoulders and a slight bend in the knees. Select a leg to begin with and gently lean forward, keeping that leg on the ground and moving the hand of the same side toward the top of the foot. Allow the other leg to lift as your upper body moves forward, keeping it on the same plane as your upper body (when your upper body is parallel to the floor, your opposite leg should be as well). When you have bent as far as is comfortable and feel your hamstrings flex, pause briefly and return to your starting position. Complete your set with each individual leg before switching sides.

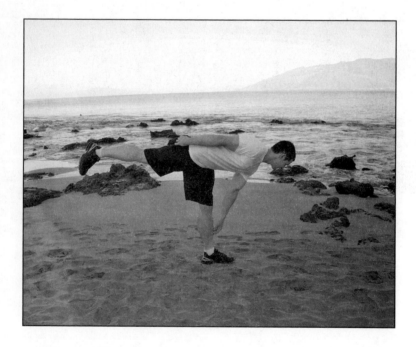

Roman Deadlift

Take two equally weighted objects in your hands and keep the hands just in front of your thighs as you stand tall with a slight bend in your knees. Keeping your back straight and your weight over your hips, lean forward, keeping the weights as close to your legs as possible as you descend. Pause when you just about reach your feet and return to the standing position.

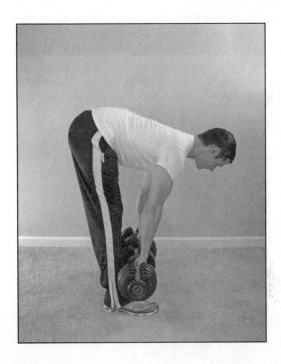

One-Leg Squat

Few exercises are as impressive as a properly conducted one-leg squat. Some of the best athletes in the world are unable to do even a single rep of this exercise, let alone a full set. In time, though, you'll not only be able to do these, you'll be the envy of your friends with a pair of muscular legs to go along with it.

Stand with your knees slightly bent and your arms straight out in front of you (this is to act as a counterbalance). Lift one leg off the ground and place it as far out in front of you as possible while keeping it straight (don't worry, you'll get better in time). Then, slowly lower yourself as far as possible on your balancing leg. When your hamstring touches your calf (or as far as you can go in the beginning stages), push yourself back up to the starting position.

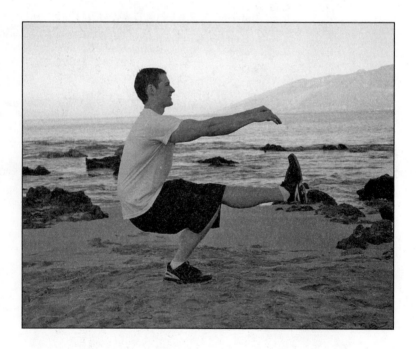

V Dips

Make your body into a V-like shape by leaning forward and placing your hands flat on the ground and placing your legs behind you enough so that you are up on the balls of your feet. From here, bend and dip your knees forward until they are just off the ground, and then return to full extension, staying on your toes the entire repetition.

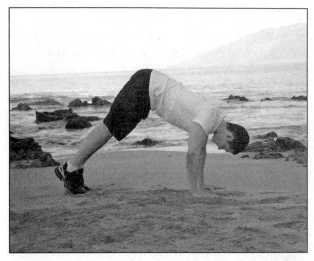

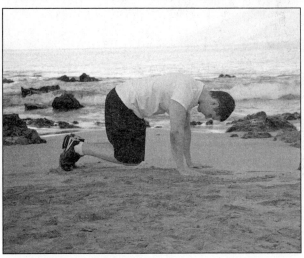

Wall Squats

Place your back against a flat, smooth wall and set your feet out slightly in front of you. Slide yourself down the wall until your hips pass slightly below your knees and then push against the bottoms of your feet until you return to the top.

Ripped addition: Prop yourself up on the balls of your feet while doing these squats.

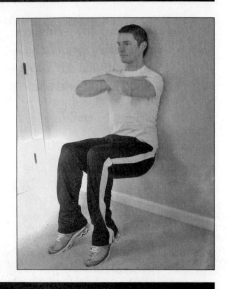

Wall Sits

This is just like a wall squat, only you hold your lowered stance for a set period of time. Start with repeats of 20-second holds and increase as able.

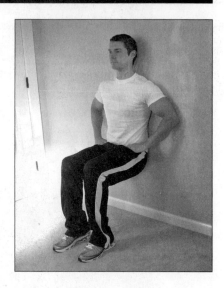

Front Kicks

For this quadriceps-strengthening exercise, stand straight up with your legs in line with your body. Place your hands on your hips and raise one leg, bent at the knee, until your quadriceps is parallel to the floor. Then, extend the leg from the knee down until it is straight in front of you. Bend back to the raised position, then lower the leg. To work your balance, don't allow your foot to touch the floor in between repetitions.

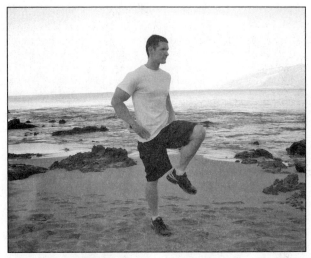

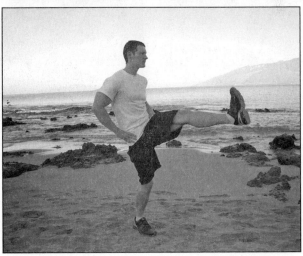

Chair Squats

You can do this with a chair or any other solid surface about the same height. Start standing in front of the object, facing away from it, and slowly lower yourself onto it in a seated position. Then, try to return to the standing position while keeping your back as straight as possible.

Ripped addition: Do it with just one leg!

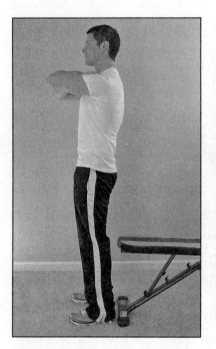 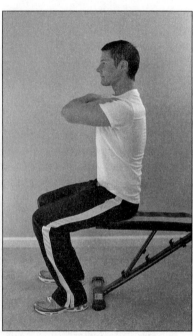

Standing Rear Leg Extensions

Standing up straight, place your hands on your hips. Select a leg to start with and raise it slightly off the ground. While maintaining as upright a posture as possible, draw the leg up behind you as high as possible with your toes pointed.

Ripped addition: Start in a push-up position with your feet elevated to nearly the same height, or the same height, as your upper body. Raise one leg at a time as high as possible.

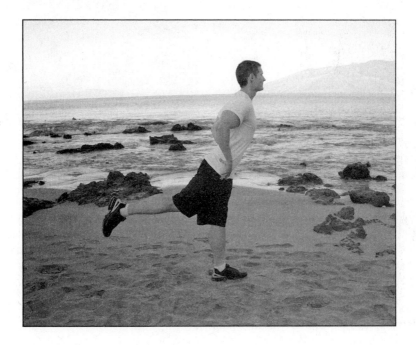

Standing Side Leg Extensions

From a standing position with your legs in line with your body, shift your weight onto one leg and lift the other out to the side as high as possible. Return to the starting position. Try not to allow your active leg to touch the ground in between repetitions.

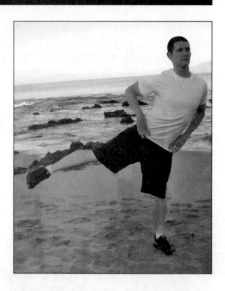

Hip Lifts

Lie on your side propped up on an elbow and with your legs extended and on top of one another. Lift your top leg while keeping it in line with the leg that is remaining stationary. Pause when you reach the height of your ability and then lower your leg back *near* your starting position. During the course of your set, don't allow your feet or ankles to touch and always keep your active leg hovering above the stationary one in between reps.

Ripped addition: Use an exercise cord or an ankle weight to add tension and increase the difficulty of this exercise.

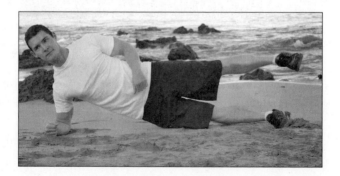

One-Leg Hip Lifts

Lie on your back with one leg bent and your knee pointing upward. Set the ankle of your opposite leg above the knee of the bent leg so that your knee is pointing out toward the side. Drive down with the foot on the ground, lifting your hips as high as possible. Pause at the top before lowering yourself nearly to the starting position, but remaining just a bit off the ground.

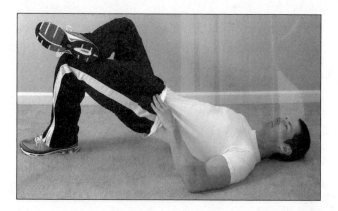

Hamstring Leg Raise

Lie with your stomach on the floor and prop yourself up on your elbows and one knee. Extend the opposite leg, point your toe, and lift the leg skyward as high as possible.

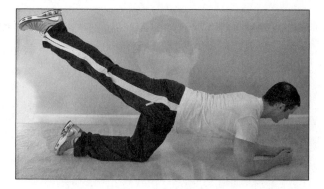

Reverse Leg-ups

Start lying face down on the floor with your arms bent out in front of you or crossed over one another. Point your toes and lift your legs as high as possible.

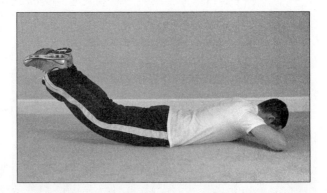

Rocking Push-ups

Start with your feet in the traditional push-up position but your upper body balancing on your elbows and forearms with your palms flat on the floor. Maintaining your arms in their current position, use your hamstrings and arms to create a 'V' shape with your body, lifting your hips as high as you can. Slowly return to the starting position.

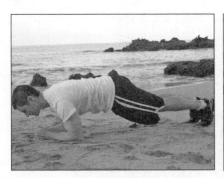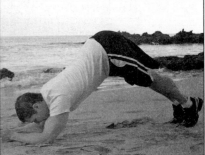

Merry-Go-Round

Stand up with your feet spread apart comfortably. With your arms extended and palms open, lean down so that your hands are touching the outside of your left ankle. Now in a rainbow-like motion, slowly raise your arms up above and over your body until they assume the same position outside of your right ankle. Repeat back and forth.

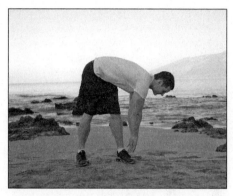

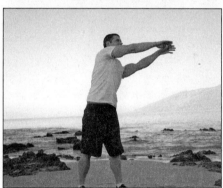

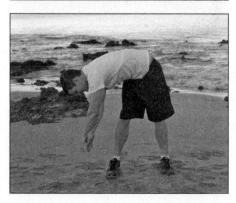

Cable Squats

Standing on your stretch cord, squat down and grab an end of the cord in each hand, giving yourself a small bit of slack. Now stand up slowly, pushing through the added resistance of the stretching cable.

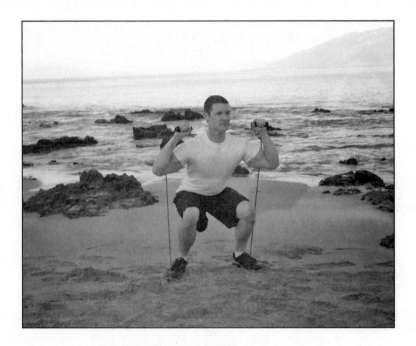

Box Jumps

Find a stable bench or other solid platform that is within reasonable jumping height. From a standing position with your feet shoulder-width apart, bend slightly at the knees and leap onto the platform and immediately back off. Repeat for repetitions.

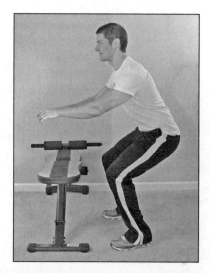

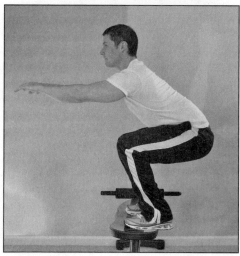

Knee-High Jumps

Stand tall and spread your feet slightly apart. Bend at the knees and leap into the air as high as you can, drawing your knees upward as you go. On the downward position of the jump, ensure you have extended your legs again—maintaining a comfortable bend—and land carefully on the balls of your feet. Repeat for repetitions.

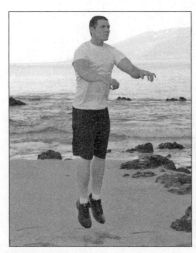 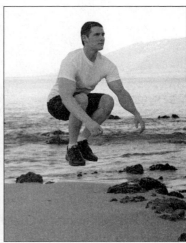

Fitness Ball Squat

Place a fitness ball between your back and a wall and lower yourself into a seated position. Pause when your quadriceps are parallel to the floor and then raise yourself back up.

Variation: Do each squat with just one leg at a time.

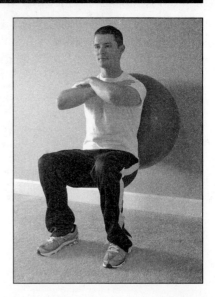

Fitness Ball Hamstring Curls

Lie on the floor on your back with your feet on a fitness ball and your hips elevated from the floor. Bending at the knees, draw the ball toward you as far as you can and back out to the starting position.

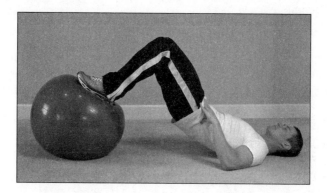

Calves

Calves are generally an afterthought when it comes to training, but real athletes and fitness enthusiasts know they can't be neglected. Think about it; any good building has to have a solid foundation. Your body is no different. The calves—mostly made up of the Soleus and the Gastroc-nemius muscles—are the first major muscles that form your base. Don't neglect them! While the calves are a muscle that is often very genetically based—in that some people can't make them grow very large no matter what they do and others don't do anything and have huge calves—they're still important. After all, you can't build a big house on weak beams, but you can build your dream on strong ones.

Calf Raises

Stand facing a stair (you don't need a staircase, even just one small ledge works for this). Step onto the platform with the balls of your feet on the edge of the step and the remainder of your foot and heel hanging over the edge above the ground. Slowly lower yourself so your heels are below the step, then lift yourself on the balls of your feet as high as possible. Pause at the top, lower slowly, and repeat.

Ripped addition: To increase variety and create a more complete feeling that you've worked both major muscles in the calves (the Gastrocnemius and Soleus), you can also turn your toes out for several sets, and then in for several sets.

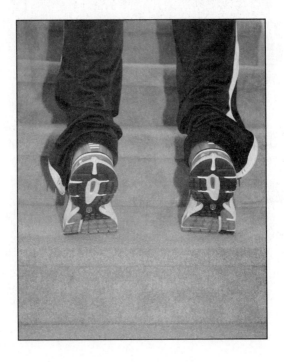

One-Leg Calf Raise

Assume the same position as you would in the prior exercise, but rather than having both feet on the edge of the step, place the top of one foot behind the ankle of the other, leaving you balancing on one foot. In the same fashion as with both feet, slowly lower yourself down as far as you comfortably can go, and then lift yourself up as high as possible onto the ball of the foot, pausing at the top before repeating.

Ripped addition: You can use the same variations with one-leg raises as you can with the two-leg version of this exercise.

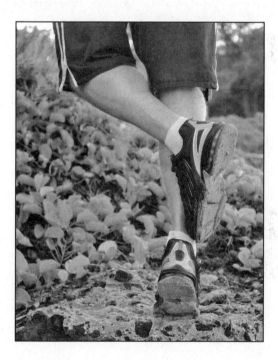

Core Exercises and Full Body Fun

You can follow a strict diet and burn away all the body fat you want, but the bottom line is if you want ripped abs, you have to have some muscle to show once the top layers have been "removed," so to speak. Getting that much-desired six pack requires diligence in the kitchen, but also with your core training. And strengthening your abdominals and lower back muscles also makes everything from sitting to standing, walking to running, easier and more comfortable.

Traditional Crunch

Cross your arms over your chest (*not* behind your head). This is your traditional, old-school crunch. The thing to focus on here is to raise your body *up* and not *forward,* which is where most people go wrong with this exercise.

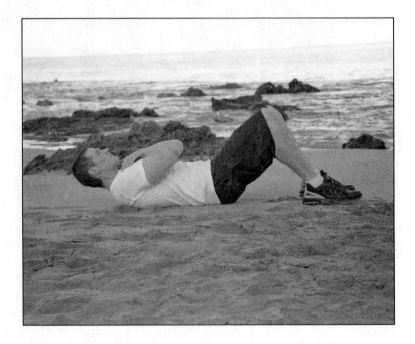

Oblique Twist

With your feet securely under a solid object to hold your lower body steady, lift your body *upward* until your back is just off the ground and extend your arms out to their respective sides. Start rotating to one side, bringing with you the arm from the side you're turning away from. Rotate your core until that hand touches the other hand, which should remain in place. Return to your starting position and rotate to the opposite side.

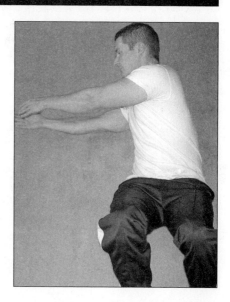

Elbow Hold

Place your body and feet facing down as if you are going to do a traditional push-up, but prop yourself up on your elbows instead. Your elbows should be under your chest, and your hands should be pointing forward, ending up under your face. Hold this position for varied amounts of time. If you're new to training, start with 15 to 20 seconds and increase incrementally as you improve.

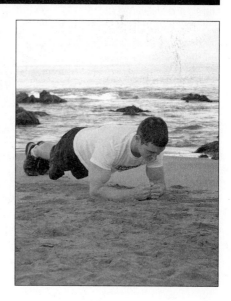

Push-up Hold

Extend your arms to the beginning position of a traditional push-up. Position your feet a bit wider than usual and draw one arm back or place one hand on your hip. Hold this position starting with 15 to 20 seconds as you begin, and increase over time.

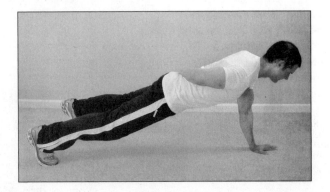

Knee-ups on Doorframe

Using a doorframe or another elevated object you can hang from, allow yourself to remain suspended at arms' length. Lift your legs as high as possible in front of you before lowering them.

Ripped addition: You can do these in a trio of positions. First, raise your legs as high as possible to the left, return to starting position, then raise to center, return to starting position, then raise to the right.

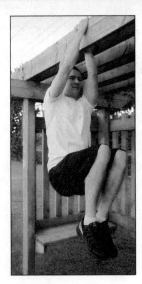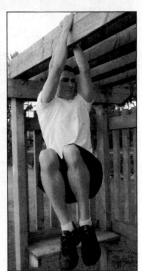

Side Plank

Lie on the floor on your side and prop yourself up so that only your forearm is on the ground. Place your legs atop one another and lift yourself up so that you are in a straight line from the feet all the way up your body. As with the elbow and push-up holds, start with brief holds of 15 to 20 seconds and increase the amount of time as you get stronger. Alternate sides for equal lengths of time.

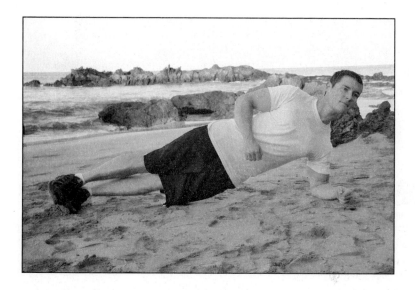

Abdominal Flutter Kick

Lie on the floor flat on your back and place your hands, palms down, beneath your butt. Lift your heels slightly off the ground and point your toes. Kick your legs up and down slightly as if you are swimming.

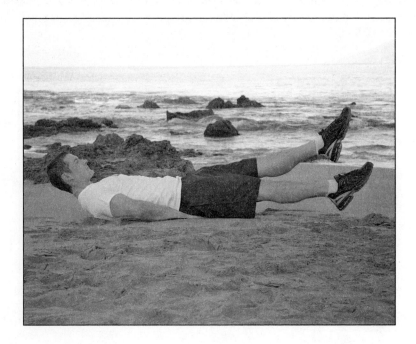

Abdominal Leg Raises

Lie on the floor flat on your back and bring your heels off the ground. If you find it more comfortable, you may place your hands beneath your lower back or butt. Raise your legs until you feel the whole of your abdominals contracting, then lower them to the starting position. Never allow your heels to touch the ground during this exercise.

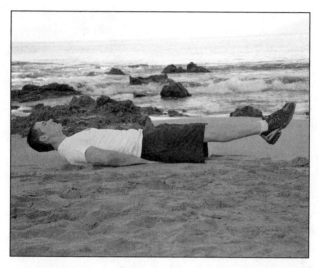

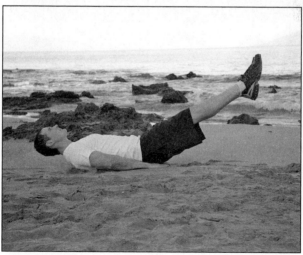

V-ups

Lie on the floor on your back with your body fully extended, with your legs straight and your arms also extended above you. Now, lift your legs at the same time as you lift your upper body and arms and touch your hands to your toes (or get as close as possible).

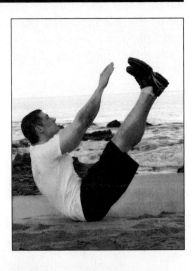

Fitness Ball Ab Walk

Start with your hands flat on the floor and your knees on a fitness ball. Slowly walk yourself out with your hands until your back is flat.

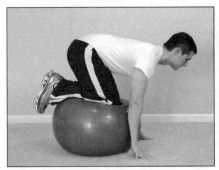 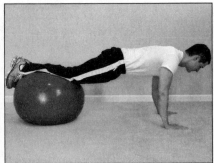

Fitness Ball Crunch

Sit on a fitness ball and move your feet forward until your lower back is positioned evenly on the ball. Cross your arms over your chest or place them behind your head and crunch, focusing on moving *up* and not *forward* with your body.

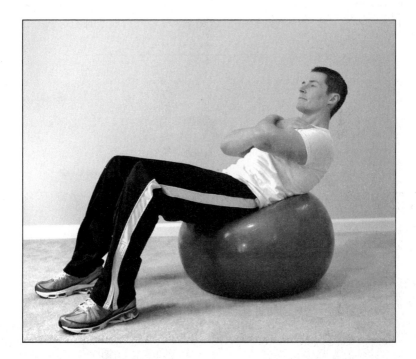

Good Mornings

This is a great exercise for your lower back.

Stand up tall with your legs nearly straight and bend your elbows to place your hands behind your head, interlocking your fingers. Bending only at the waist, lean forward until your upper body becomes flat. Pause in that position just briefly before slowly returning to your starting position.

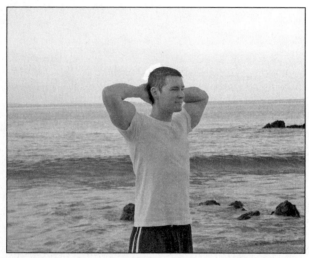

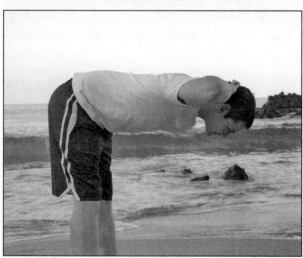

Full Bridge

With your back on the floor, bend at the knees until your feet are flat on the ground. Place your arms so that your elbows are pointing to the ceiling and your palms are flat on either side of your head. In one smooth motion, push from your palms and heels and lift yourself off the ground.

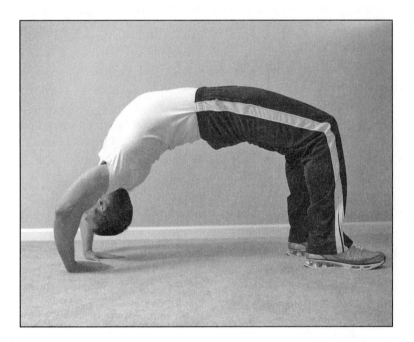

Hands-Under-Butt Bridge

Lie on your back with your hands under your butt and your knees bent up so that your feet are flat on the floor and positioned just outside of your shoulders. Push from the bottoms of your hands and feet until your hips are lifted as high as possible. Hold briefly in this position and return to the starting position.

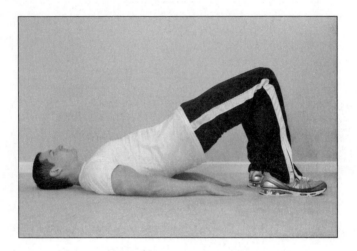

Ripped alternative: Do the same exercise using only one leg.

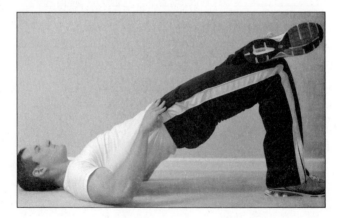

Overhead Leg Extensions

From the floor, roll onto your back until your legs are hanging over your head. Keep your arms extended down the length of your body and flat. Using your core, extend your legs straight above you as you try to position your torso as vertical as possible.

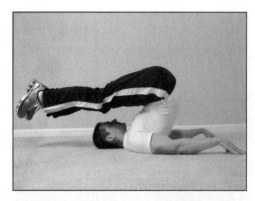

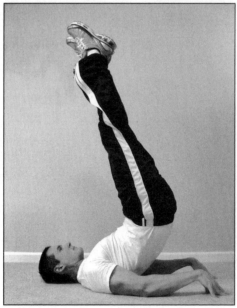

Overhead Towers

Sit on the floor and roll backward until your knees are above your face. Place your elbows on the ground at your sides and your hands lightly on your lower back. Extend the body as if you're trying to touch your pointed toes to the ceiling, then slowly lower back to the starting position.

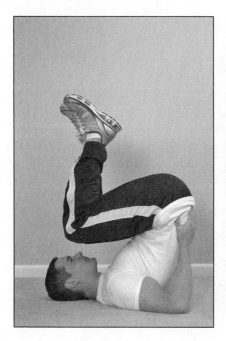
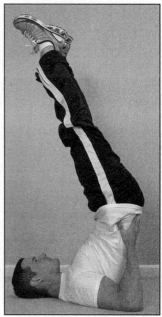

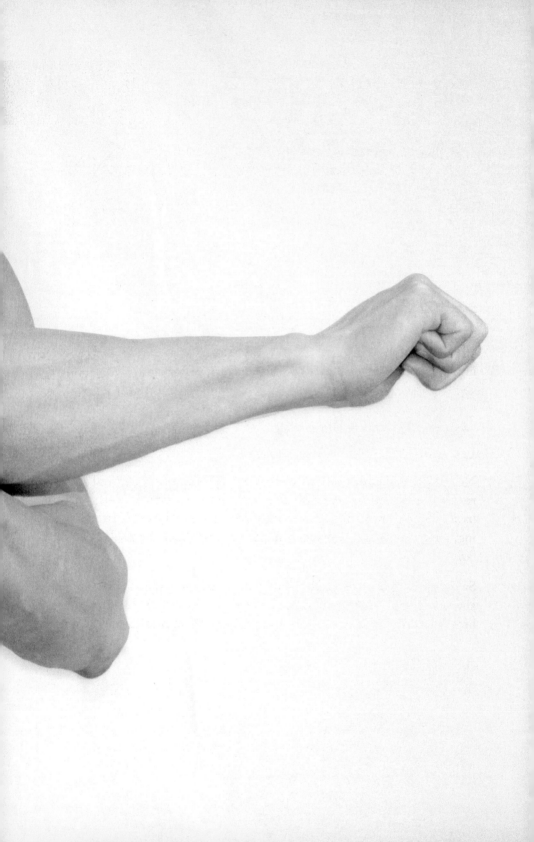

4

Longer, Leaner Muscles

Although stretching is not often seen as traditional "exercise," it's a fantastic way to train your muscles. The benefits of stretching include increased comfort, mobility, and range of motion, as well as reduced risk of injury. And best of all, a complete stretching session takes only minutes and requires no accessories.

Understanding Stretching

Not all stretching is created equal, and while it isn't necessary to have read a dissertation on each type that's out there, it's worth knowing the basics for your own safety. There are seven different "types" of stretching, some that should be avoided and others that should be used regularly.

Safe stretching involves getting into your stretching position comfortably and holding that position while breathing regularly. Don't hold your breath and don't force a muscle past a comfortable stretching point.

Active Isolated Stretching

Active isolated stretching is very common to activities like yoga. The premise is that when a muscle contracts as it's isolated, the opposite muscle will relax. Sometimes getting into position for these types of stretches can be difficult, making this type of training relatively uncommon for most people.

Ballistic Stretching

Ballistic stretching is also known as "bad stretching" in a lot of training circles. The ideology behind this type of stretching involves overstretching a muscle by exerting force or using momentum such as bouncing. As you can tell just by the description, this goes against the "slow-and-hold" method we encourage with stretching.

Dynamic Stretching

Dynamic stretching is a better form of the techniques used in ballistic stretching. While it also uses movement to stretch the muscles, it avoids the bouncing or abrupt end of the stretch where injury can occur. Circling your arms or taking deep steps (like lunges) are examples of dynamic stretching.

Isometric Stretching

Even those who don't know anything about exercise tend to do isometric stretching. Isometric stretches involve other objects (which can be furniture, walls, or even people) that you can move the body against to increase tension and thus develop flexibility. For example, if you lift your foot and place your toes against the lower portion of a wall and gently lean into it and hold that position, you will feel your calves stretch. This is an isometric stretch.

Passive Stretching

Passive stretching may also be called "relaxed" stretching. It involves using an apparatus of sorts—which can be another person, a solid object, or another part of your body—to apply and hold the stretched position and, if necessary, increase pressure for you.

PNF Stretching

The long-winded name for PNF stretching is proprioceptive neuromuscular facilitation stretching, which is a mixture of stretching techniques originally designed for use in rehabilitation training. These types of stretches look to increase flexibility through a muscle's entire range of motion. PNF stretching requires someone, generally a practicing thera-pist, to lead the subject through the various techniques.

Static Stretching

The most basic and most common type of stretching is called static stretching. This means it's without motion, so once you get yourself into position, you simply hold it for the duration of your stretch.

Static stretching is sometimes confused with passive stretching, as the two tend to share characteristics and are in fact similar. Whereas passive stretching involves increasing the stretch or further involving a muscle into a stretch, static stretching lengthens a muscle and then holds it in one position.

The Rules of Stretching

To get the most out of your stretches and to keep them safe, follow these basic guidelines:

Stop if it hurts. Stretching should be relaxing and used to increase your circulation and flexibility. If you feel pain while you are stretching, you're doing something wrong—either stretching too far or aren't warmed up enough yet. If you feel pain, stop and reassess.

Don't allow momentum to influence your stretch. With whatever stretch you're doing, slowly find the point at which you feel adequate tension and hold there. Never "fall into" a stretch or "bounce" to get fur-ther. Go to where it feels good, and hold.

Hold each stretch for at least 30 seconds. Doing so allows the muscles and surrounding tissue to become accustomed to the expanded range of motion. If you don't hold a stretch long enough, the body won't adapt and you won't see much benefit from your efforts.

Always breathe. It's natural to try to hold your breath particularly dur-ing some of the more unusual stretches, but you don't want to do that. Breathe fully and deeply and relax.

Ultimate Stretches

Stretches don't have to be complicated to serve their purpose. And you don't have to go to extraordinary lengths to start getting the benefits from stretching. In fact, within days after starting these stretches, you'll find yourself feeling much more limber and you'll note progress at a pretty rapid pace. Don't worry if you can't stretch very far in any one position; you'll get there soon enough.

Upper Body Stretches

Most people work out after work. But so many people use the excuse "I'm tired," to avoid doing it, or come up with something like "I don't feel well, I have a headache." That's because many people work in jobs that don't involve much movement—such as sitting at a desk all day—and they really do leave the office feeling tired, sore, or in some sort of pain. A lot of people have headaches at the end of the workday, and you might be surprised to know it isn't just from your boss: It's more likely due to tight muscles.

Muscles connect with one another throughout the body, and one tight group can affect your overall well-being. Your hamstrings, for instance, can be a large cause of pain in the lower back. Similarly, tight muscles in the back and shoulders can cause neck pain (on top of your neck muscles also potentially being tight), which leads to headaches. As you can tell, it's a vicious cycle, and one you can fix immediately with some quality stretching.

Chest—Wall Stretch

Face a wall or other solid and sturdy object and extend an arm against it. Your palm should be open and flat against the object. Keep your arm in this position and slowly turn your body away from the wall until you feel your chest stretch. Maintain this position until you are ready to switch sides, then simply switch arms.

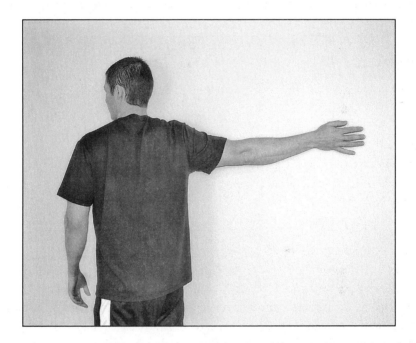

Chest—Corner Stretch

You can use any corner of a room for this stretch as long as the walls on either side of you are flat and sturdy. Place yourself so that you are looking right into the corner where the walls come together. Put one hand on each wall just above head level with your palms open. Slowly lean forward into the corner until you feel your chest stretch and hold that position. Alternatively, you may use a doorframe to achieve a similar stretch.

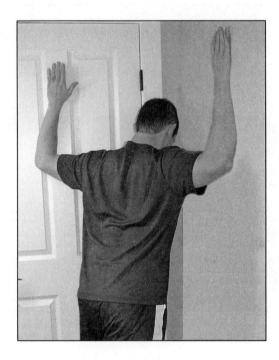

Chest—Platform Stretch

Kneel down facing a chair (preferably one without arms). Place your elbows on the edges of the seat and fold your arms down toward the middle on top of one another. Ensure your knees are far enough back that as you lean forward, your head passes in front of the chair. Lean until you feel your pectorals stretch.

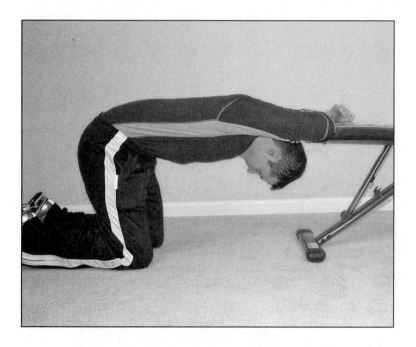

Biceps—Door Stretch

Stand with your back to an open door and reach back with the appropriate arm to grasp the edge, doing so with your thumb pointing down. Slide your arm up behind you until you feel your biceps stretch.

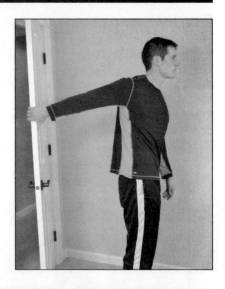

Triceps—Bent Arm Stretch

Raise an arm straight above you and bend at the elbow as if you are going to pat yourself on the back, ensuring the elbow itself does not move. Using your opposite hand, reach up and over and pull gently on the outside of your elbow to create the stretch.

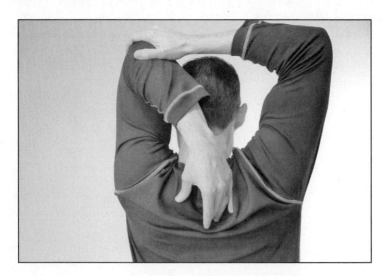

Triceps—Door Stretch

Open a door and face the edge. Bring an arm above you, bent at the elbow, and place the underside of your upper arm on the side of the door. Lean your body forward to create the stretch (feel free to use your foot and other hand to steady the door if necessary).

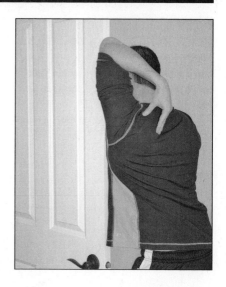

Forearms—Press Stretch

This simple stretch is very useful for grip strength and comfort. Simply take one hand and press back against the extended fingers of the other hand. Gently press back until you feel your forearm stretch, hold this position for the duration of the exercise, and then rotate.

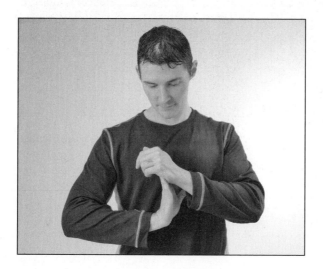

Forearms—Seated Stretch

From a seated position on the floor, sit with your back straight and your arms straight down at your sides with the palms open and touching the floor and your fingers out front. Keeping your arms close to your body, slowly lean forward while ensuring that your palms maintain contact with the floor. You should feel the stretch slowly extended throughout your forearms.

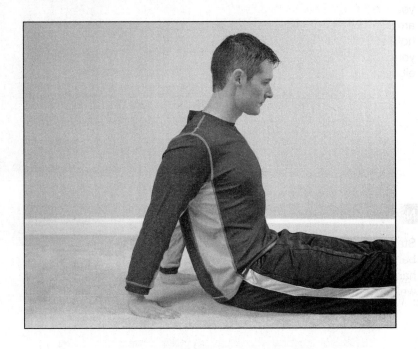

Shoulder—Rail Stretch

Start with either arm and find a handle or other solid object you can grip
that is just above waist high (a stair
railing may be perfect, for instance).
Keeping your elbow stationary at
your side, bend your arm (so your
arm will be in an "L" shape) and grab
hold of the railing/handle. Slowly turn
your body out while keeping your
elbow at your side.

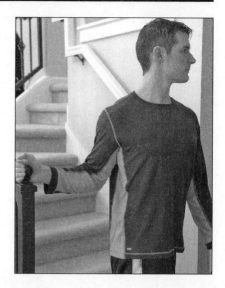

Neck—Behind Back Stretch

Stand up straight and relaxed. Use one hand to grasp the opposite wrist
behind your back. Now, slowly lean your neck to the side of the grasping
hand while using your grip to ensure that your shoulders do not come up as
well. Hold the stretch and then rotate positions.

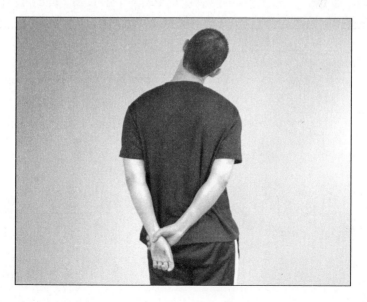

Neck—Floor Stretch

Lie on your back with your knees bent and feet flat on the floor. With both hands, gently grip behind your head and press your face in the direction of your knees without allowing any other part of your body to move.

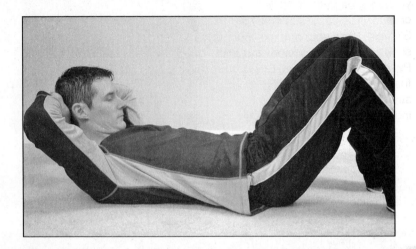

Posterior Neck—Roll Over Stretch

Lie on your back and raise your legs off the floor and over your head until they are past your shoulders. Use your hands on your back to help support the body and try to bring your feet to the floor.

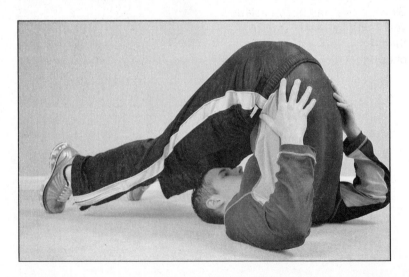

Back and Core—Streamline Stretch

This is a great stretch for your core and back. Extend your arms straight above your head, cover your ears with your biceps, and cross one hand over the other. Slowly lean to one side and feel the stretch in your opposite lat muscle. Pause and hold in this position before leaning to the other side. This stretch can also be done while lying on your back.

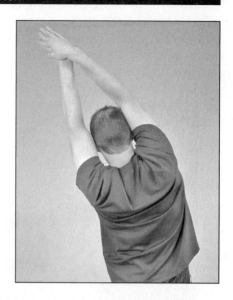

Back—Wall Stretch

Facing a wall, put both of your palms flat on the wall just about shoulder-width apart and slide your hands so that they are about one to two feet above your head. Slowly move your body back until your arms are nearly straight and then simply lean your head and chest forward between your arms.

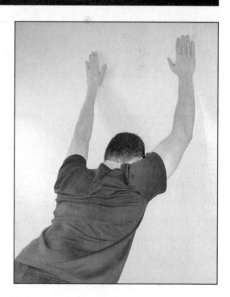

Back—Rail Stretch

Keep a slight bend in your knees and grab a vertical pole or railing (if necessary you can also use door handles). Position your body so that your back is nearly flat and slowly allow your body to lean back while exhaling until you feel your back muscles stretch.

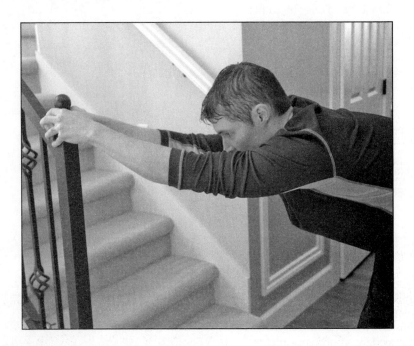

Core Stretches

Your abdominals and lumbar regions are vastly important to the overall structure of your body. These areas are associated with the term "core," and should be trained—and stretched—with the same diligence as other muscle groups. Doing so will ensure everything from bending over to pick something up, to even standing with proper posture, is much easier and more comfortable.

Cobra Stretch

From the ground, face down with your stomach on the floor. From here, slowly push yourself up with your arms; once you begin to feel a stretch in your core, hold that position. Throughout this stretch do not involve your lower body.

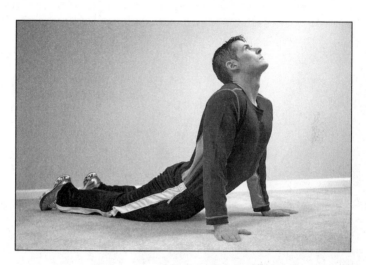

Obliques—Lean Stretch

Stand up tall and relaxed with your arms at your sides and slowly lean to one side until you feel a stretch in your side. You can also do this stretch by raising and reaching over yourself with the arm on the side of the body you are stretching.

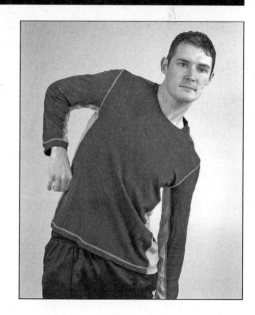

Lower Back—Chair Stretch

Sit in a chair with a flat bottom and place your feet out flat in front of you. Scoot yourself forward until you are near the end of the seat. Move your feet so that they are beyond shoulder-width and place your hands on your calves. Lean forward slowly and, as you do, slide your hands down until they are behind your ankles. You may press your upper body against your legs as you go to increase the stretch in your lower back.

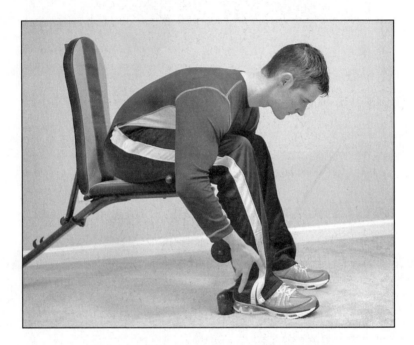

Lower Body Stretches

As I mentioned at the beginning of this chapter, tight hamstrings can cause pain in your back as well as your legs. Likewise, having tight calves and quadriceps can make the world's simplest form of exercise—walking—painful and uncomfortable. Your legs and hips are involved in everything you do. Even if you are training your upper body, you have to be balanced on your legs, and ensuring they are well trained and flexible makes everything you do easier and safer.

Quadriceps—Standing Stretch

Bend at the knee and bring a heel toward your butt. Use the hand on that side of the body and gently pull back on your toes until you feel your quadriceps stretch. Do the same thing with the other leg.

You may find that your balance isn't developed enough yet to do this stretch free-standing, so feel free to hold on to a chair, wall, or partner while doing this stretch.

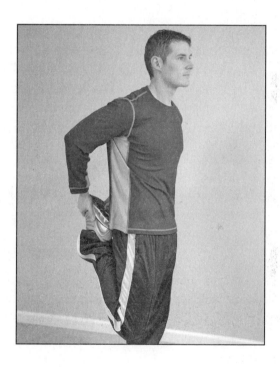

Quadriceps—Floor Stretch

Sit on the floor with your legs extended out in front of you. Select a leg to start with and bend at that knee, placing the top of the foot on the floor underneath your butt or, if it's more comfortable, next to your hip. Slowly lean backward until you feel your quadriceps begin to stretch, hold there, and then alternate legs.

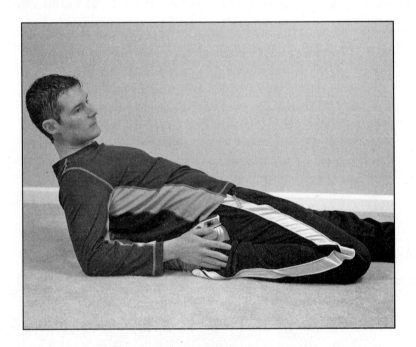

Hamstrings—Lean Stretch

Sit on the ground with your legs out in front of you and slowly lean forward, running your open palms down the front of your legs until you feel your hamstrings begin to stretch. Pause at that position, hold for several seconds, and try to extend further down your leg if possible. When you are as far as you can comfortably go, hold that position. Make sure you are breathing easily and fluidly, as holding your breath will compromise the stretch.

It is also important with this stretch to be very aware of your body movement so that you do not bounce up and down. For many years this stretch was taught with that very bouncing movement, but this can be dangerous and should be avoided.

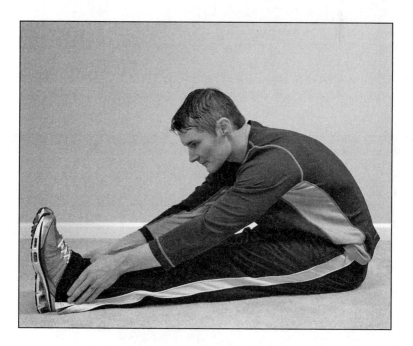

Hamstring—Bench Stretch

Set your leg straight out on a solid object that is a comfortable height and gently lean forward, keeping your leg that is still in contact with the ground at a slight bend. You may also do a variation of this from the ground, with both legs.

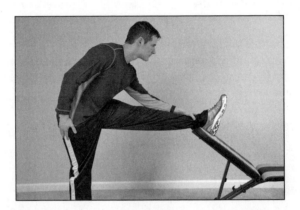

Hamstring and Glutes Stretch

Lie on a flat surface on your back with one leg on the platform with you and the other hanging off. Using both hands, draw the leg on the platform up to your chest by bending at the knee and holding it upward to create the stretch.

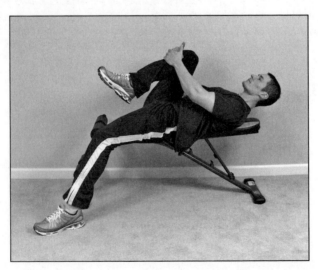

Hips—Cross Stretch

Start relaxed on the ground lying on your back. Select a leg and bend at the knee, bringing it up as if toward your chest. When it is as close to your chest as is comfortable, cross it over your body and onto the ground while keeping your back flat. Exhale fully and allow your body to relax into the stretch, then repeat with the other leg.

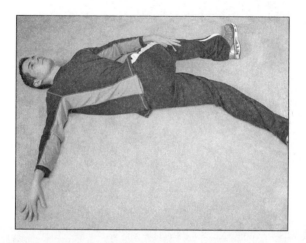

Groin—Butterfly Stretch

Sit on the floor with your heels in toward the body and the bottoms of your feet touching. Your knees will be pointing out to each side. Place your hands over your ankles and use your elbows to gently and very slowly press down against the insides of your knees.

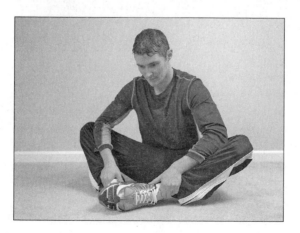

Groin and Hamstrings—Forward Lean Stretch

Sit on the floor and place your legs as far out to the sides as possible while keeping your legs straight. Slowly lean forward.

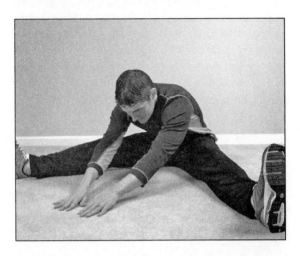

Calves—Wall Stretch

Place your hands on a wall with a bend in your arms. Select a foot and slowly slide it straight behind you, allowing your opposite knee to bend as necessary while you do. Ensure your heel stays flat on the ground and, when you feel a stretch in your calf, pause and hold this position for your stretch. Alternate legs when ready to do so.

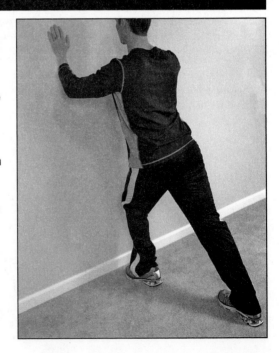

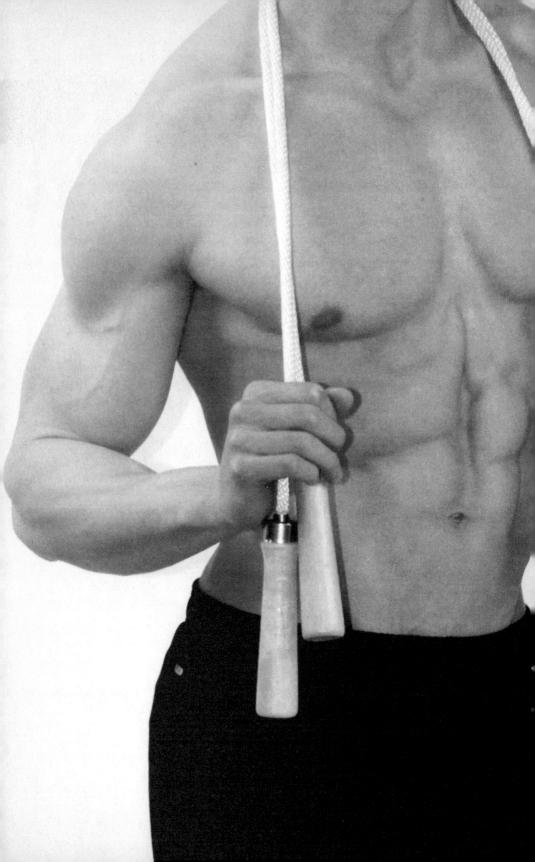

5

Cardio Exercises

There's definitely something magical about sustained aerobic exercise. The body wants you to love it so much, in fact, that as you continue on, it releases endorphins and other chemicals natural to the body to increase your mood. The body *wants* to get you hooked on heart-healthy exercise. And in addition to the fact that you'll become addicted to how good you feel, you'll experience a litany of other positive effects to go with it. After you notice increased fat loss, leaner muscles, and a healthier cardiovascular system, you'll find that this "cardio" thing is really a win-win and most definitely worth the time and effort.

An important point to remember: Cardiovascular exercise isn't the best way to burn body fat and get the body of your dreams. Building new muscle is. But that doesn't mean that cardio is without benefits or without purpose. Those extra calories you burn are definitely going to add up over time, definitely going to help you slim down to that smaller pair of jeans, and definitely going to help you live a longer life. Just don't expect miracles in the mirror if you're doing hours of cardio and nothing else. The simple fact is cardio—like any exercise—can be undone with a couple of beers, or a couple of sodas, or a big, juicy burger.

So do cardio workouts because they are fun and healthy, but don't expect miracles from cardio training if you don't stay focused on other facets of your training, such as proper diet and strength training.

Circuits to Condition the Whole Body

People who run marathons, and those brave enough to try *ultra-marathons*, deserve a great deal of admiration. Their dedication to their craft is unparalleled. On top of being able to do what seem to most people as superhuman tasks, they're also in great shape. But, that said, you don't have to do what they do—or attempt to do what they do—to get the kind of lean physique they often have.

While you can definitely put on the running shoes and go run for as many miles as you enjoy, you might find that you don't have the time to do so regularly. Or you might just be the type of person who doesn't particularly care for long runs. That's just fine, too. This chapter provides you with a variety of aerobic and anaerobic exercises designed to help you melt away annoying body fat. They don't require large chunks of time to do and they are all designed to create results that you can see in short order while keeping you entertained.

It's important to make sure that you do a variety of cardiovascular exercises to increase your heart rate and work your body. The reason for this is because of something called "adaptation." Like anything, the more you do something, the better—and thus more efficient—you become at it. When you do this, the good kind of resistance you were placing on your body becomes more and more negligible. The body doesn't have to work as hard to go through the motions, and you start working a different type of muscle fiber. In contrast, if you consistently create variety in your training, your body doesn't get used to the same motion over and over, day after day, and becomes more efficient at burning fat for fuel rather than simply more efficient with a particular movement. You get to work new energy systems while keeping the body guessing, and thus allowing yourself to continually progress.

Now, that isn't to say you can't do the same kind of cardio work two days in a row. But the more variety you can introduce into your workouts, the better. If you do three days of cardiovascular exercise each week, and if you do something different each of those three days, that's a great, varied routine. For instance, you might run on Monday, use an elliptical trainer or treadmill you may have at home on Wednesday, and do a kick-boxing type of cardio on Friday (or any variation thereof),. But if, based on your work schedule, travel, or even weather, you have to do one type of exercise for a couple of days straight, feel free. Just make sure you switch it up when it becomes possible to do so.

Need-to-Know Cardio Exercises

Some simple exercises make for exceptional cardio training. The movements described in the following sections work a variety of muscles, which is what makes them so valuable for getting your heart rate up. Some are great additions to interval training, and some are great on their own, but like everything covered thus far, they are all, first and foremost, additional tools you can make work for you.

Burpees

The funny name belies incredible results: Burpees. They're used in just about every training program you'll ever find—in the military, in martial arts, all around the world. Few exercises are so universally accepted as effective, but this one is king. It's like a total body workout in a single exercise. Start standing with your feet shoulder-width apart. Squat down quickly and put your hands on the ground just out in front of you. Support your weight on your hands and kick your feet back, putting you in the traditional "push-up position." Do a single push-up and then push off your feet to return to the squat-down position. From here you conduct the final piece, which is a vertical jump, lifting your arms straight up above you as you do. Remember that all of these pieces are done in rapid succession.

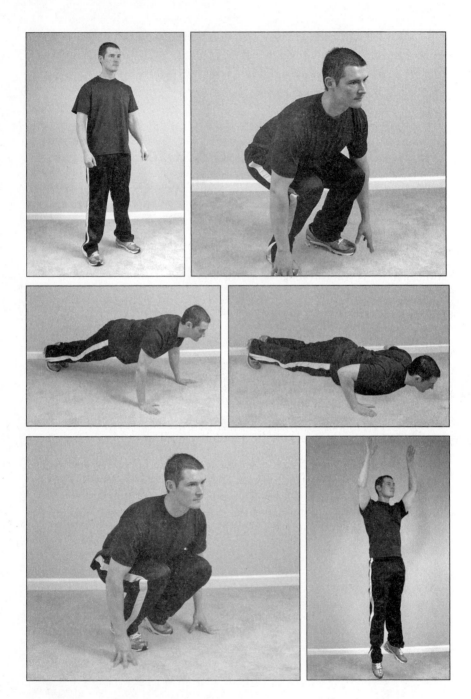

Now that you know how to do Burpees, you can put them to use.

Animal Crawls

We can take a lot from the animal kingdom when it comes to fitness. After all, the creatures in the wild have to adapt their physiologies to a myriad of terrain and obstacles. We've found over time if we mimic their motions, we can get a great workout. Here's a trio of crawls you are sure to enjoy.

Bear. Place your hands on the ground, keep your hips high, and get up on the balls of your feet. Move along the ground in this pattern which, as you'd guess, is similar to how you'd see a bear travel.

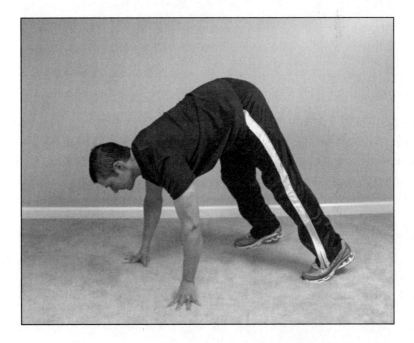

Crab. Start seated on the floor. Bend at the knees and place your feet flat on the floor. Reach behind you and place your palms on the floor as well, then lift your hips up and hold yourself off the ground. Now crawl forward and back for a set number of "laps" of your course or for a set period of time.

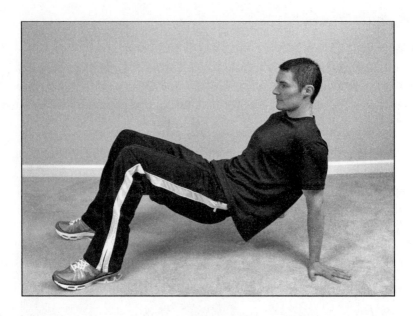

Crocodile. The "croc crawl" looks easy but it's anything but. Think of how you'd see a crocodile move over land (feel free to YouTube it if you want a real idea!) and try to do the same. Keep your body as low to the ground as possible and move one arm at the same time as the opposite leg, then move your opposite arm and leg, and see how far you can go.

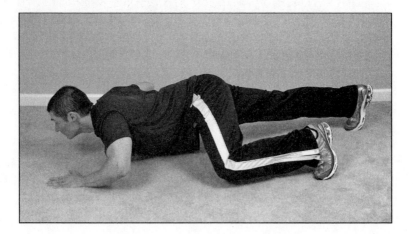

In-Home Cardio

The exercises described in this section are designed to be done indoors. While you certainly can put them to use outdoors or in a gymnasium-like setting, they're great to have in your arsenal for when the weather is bad or other facilities aren't available. That said, use them where you can and where you want to.

Mountain Climbers

Get into the traditional push-up position and then bring your hips up slightly. Alternate bringing your knees, one at a time, up to your chest. Do this quickly for a great cardiovascular workout.

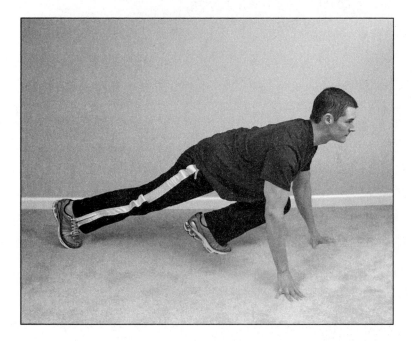

Skating

This is another fun cardiovascular exercise; the movements for this look much like a speed skater's motion. Start standing but leaning slightly forward. Balance yourself on one leg and swing both arms to one side; then hop onto the other leg while swinging your arms to the opposite side. Alternate back and forth in a smooth, steady pattern.

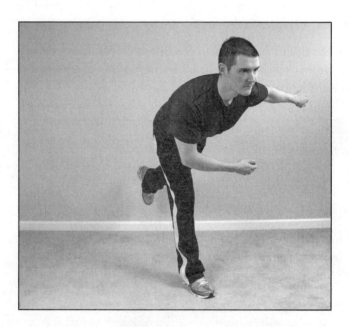

Punch Your Way to Progress

You don't have to be a well-trained fighter to use the movements that boxers and other martial arts practitioners do to get your heart rate up.

A simple, easy punch-kick combination makes for great exercise (explaining why the vast majority of fighters are in terrific shape) and many, many people find going through the motions an extremely good stress reliever. You don't have to actually hit something to release tension; just putting power into an attack motion can actually help you return to your day much more relaxed after you're done training.

Keep in mind that this exercise is for cardiovascular purposes, *not* self-defense.

Punch-Kick Combo

Take a stance that places your body in a ready position: your hands should be up and your feet just outside shoulder-width with your strong-side leg back a bit and your knees bent just slightly, remaining light on the balls of your feet. (Think of a boxer's fighting stance, and do your best imitation.)

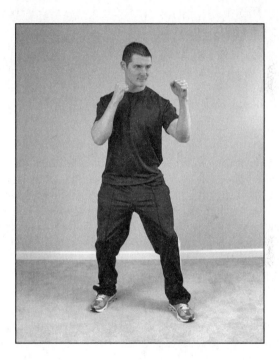

Start with a jab—a quick, short punch with your forward hand—and follow it up with a straight punch from your power hand, rotating your entire body as you throw that punch. As you return your body to the starting position from the strong hand throw, repeat the pattern. Repeat this for five rounds (for a total of ten punches).

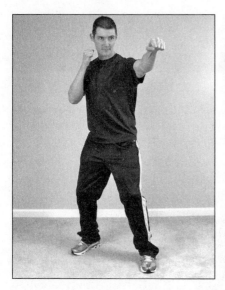
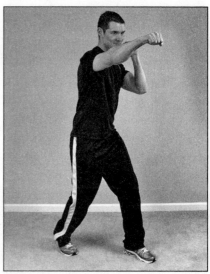

Now we get the lower body involved with front kicks. Just as with the jab, kick forward with your front leg. To do this, shift your body weight to your back leg while lifting your front knee straight up, and then flicking the lower part of your leg forward. If you were kicking a real object, you would pull your toes back as you kick so that the ball of your foot is striking the target. After that kick, place your foot down and use the same technique for your other leg. You can do this as you walk forward or, if space limits you, do so in place by simply returning each foot to the starting point. Alternate kicks until you've done a total of 10.

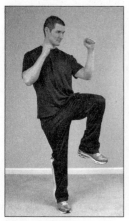
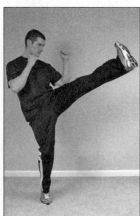
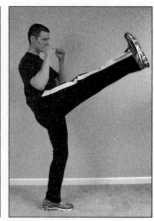

Finally, to ensure you're activating a lot of muscles in the body, return to your starting stance and add in some hooks. Starting again with your front hand, throw a hook punch just like a boxer and then return that hand as your rear (strong) hand also throws a hook. Repeat this also for a total of 10 punches.

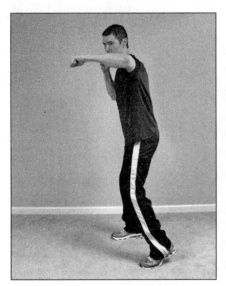 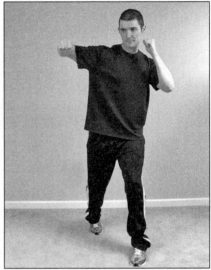

In the end, your pattern will look like this: 10 Jab/Straights, 10 Front Kicks, 10 Hooks.

When doing this for cardio, simply repeat the process as soon as you finish one rotation. If you're new, try to repeat it just three times before taking a short break. Then add rotations as you get in better shape. You can also increase the difficulty by increasing the number of strikes in each step.

You may also enjoy creating some of your own interval-style routines with these techniques. Try this one, crafted to your own level, for example:

Start by alternating between easy jabs, straights, and kicks using a comfortable number pattern (whether that's 10, 20, or more is up to you) just to keep your body moving and heart rate up; if you have the space, feel free to move about the room as you go. Then after a set time—I suggest starting with a minute—take a solid stance and see how many total quality punches—alternating jabs and straights—you can throw in 20 seconds. Then return to the original paced motions. After another minute, repeat the 20-second speed test. Increase the length of time on each portion as you become better trained and see how quickly you work up a sweat!

Stair Intervals

For a bit of cardio that also is a great workout for your legs, you need not look too far. Just find a set of stairs—whether they're in your apartment building, out at a high school football stadium, or even in your own home. Start by walking up and down a few times for an extra bit of warm-up and then get ready to put in some good work.

When you're prepared, sprint as fast as you can up the stairs, making sure your feet touch each step as you go. When you reach the top, walk back down easily, and repeat the upward sprint.

For new trainers, you may want to extend the intervals between sprints. As such, try walking up easy, down easy, sprint up, down easy, up easy, down easy, sprint up, etc.

Outdoor Cardio and Circuits

These suggestions for cardio are geared more toward open spaces. So whether that's outdoors or just somewhere with a big open floor space, you'll want to make sure you have plenty of room.

This first set doesn't require a lot of horizontal space, just some vertical room if you've got it.

Cardio Combination 1

1. 10 Burpees
2. 20 Jab/Straights

Repeat three times before a break.

To emphasize the legs, you can make a slight change:

Cardio Combination 2

1. 10 Burpees
2. 20 Front Kicks

Repeat three times before a break

Now put it all together:

Cardio Combination 3

1. 10 Burpees
2. 20 Jab/Straights
3. 20 Front Kicks

Repeat three times before a break.

The following combination can be done in a straight line if space is available, or you can do the crawls down one direction and sprint back to where you started:

Cardio Combination 4

1. Bear Crawl 10 yards
2. Sprint 10 yards
3. Crab Crawl 10 yards
4. Sprint 10 yards

Repeat three times before a break.

Interval Sprints

Many people find walking or running for the sake of exercise tedious activities. One solution—and the best way to see results—is to mix up your walking with intervals of sprinting.

Try this: After a thorough warm-up, walk for one minute. After the minute is up, sprint as fast as you can for 10 seconds. Repeat this three times and then add a three-minute walk before repeating it once more.

As your training proceeds, increase the amount of time spent sprinting by five seconds per sprint. To inch your way up when you're ready to make some changes, you can also do a ladder of sorts that looks like this:

> 1 minute walking
>
> 10 seconds sprinting
>
> 1 minute walking
>
> 15 seconds sprinting
>
> 1 minute walking
>
> 20 seconds sprinting
>
> 3 minutes walking

Repeat as appropriate for your current training level.

Cardio Timing

A technique often employed by bodybuilders and fitness models is to do low-intensity cardio exercise first thing in the morning on an empty stomach. The reasoning behind this is that after fasting through the night, the body doesn't have carbohydrates readily available to burn as fuel and, as such, must use fat instead. If you've ever turned on the television to a bodybuilding contest or flipped through a magazine, you'll notice this has been quite effective for a number of athletes. But simply getting out of bed and putting on the jogging shoes isn't enough. You do need to take precautions to spare your precious muscle.

The human body loves to store fat. It's a survival mechanism. It hasn't been but within the last century or so that food became consistently and readily available. Whether you believe in evolution or creation, it makes no difference, because that still leaves thousands of years in which finding food was sometimes a perilous journey. In response, our bodies naturally prepare for starvation by hoarding body fat for warmth and fuel. In turn, carbohydrates are burned as fuel when available and lean tissue—our muscle—is also a suitable source of energy when necessary. Both carbs and muscle are preferentially burned compared to fat. We can help to blunt this response, though, by preparing our bodies with amino acids, which are the "building blocks" of protein. Consuming a serving or two of a no-calorie amino acid supplement will help preserve your hard-earned muscle tissue while encouraging the body to burn fat.

If you want to do morning cardio, remember that low intensity (walking, jogging, treadmill, elliptical, your choice), which you will see when workouts are provided for you in Chapter 7, is different from the interval and high-intensity sets shared there.

Give this technique a try in the morning a couple of days each week and see how it works for you. Likely, you'll also find that it helps start your day off right and gives you more energy right out of the gate.

Unconventional Cardio

A cardio workout doesn't have to consist of running or aerobics. In fact, it doesn't even have to be any of the movements described in this chapter. There are things you can do throughout your day that make for great cardio exercise, and most of them don't even feel like training, which means you're more likely to do them often and for longer durations. And all that, of course, leads up to more calories burned and more fat lost. Here are just 10 suggestions for other ways to have fun and burn calories while getting a good cardio workout:

- Bicycling

- Playing basketball

- Dancing

- Hiking

- Ice skating

- Playing racquetball/squash

- Roller blading/roller skating

- Swimming

- Playing tennis

- Walking your pet

Mentally, cardio is also great for the rest of your program because it puts sweat equity into what you're doing. You know how much effort it takes to reach your goals, and by doing cardio you're giving yourself a reminder about your overall targets. After a good sweat, it's much easier to think, "If I eat junk, I'm going to waste all of this hard work."

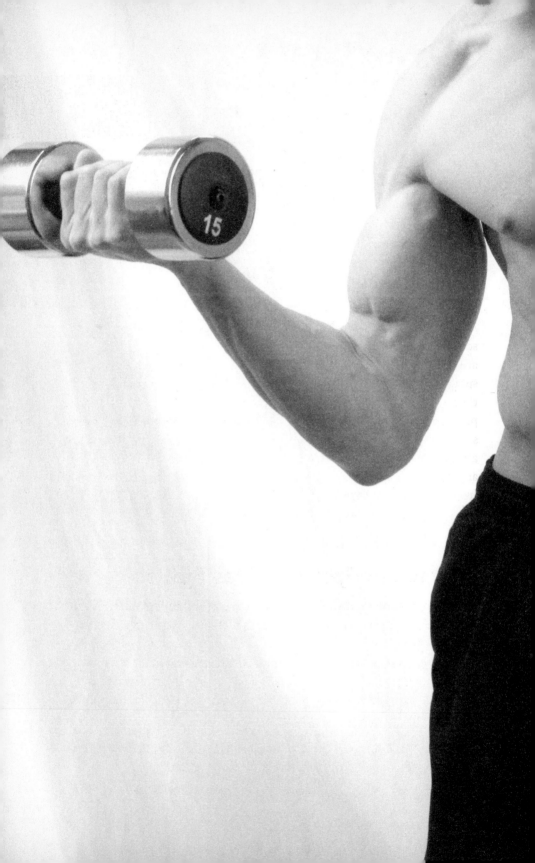

6

Creating Your Routine

A lot of books and other fitness resources think they can just throw a schedule out at you and you will somehow be able to manage your day around it. The real world just doesn't work that way. Between your job, spouse, kids, eating, sleeping, bathing, and only-you-know-what-else, there's not a lot of time for much else. Trying to squeeze in a rigid fitness program just doesn't work. Instead, what's best for *you* is to learn how to set up your own routine to fit your week. That's the only way you will be able to stick with it, see the results you want, and achieve the fitness level and body of your dreams. That's one of the reasons we train from home: It's more convenient, saves time and, oh yeah, saves money, too! Let's take a look at that before we move on.

How to Set Up: 3/4/5-Day Splits

For our purposes, we divide the body into several training areas: Shoulders, Back, Chest, Arms (Biceps/Triceps), Core, and Legs. In a perfect world you would be able to train one area per day, eat your meals at equally separated times, and get adequate rest each and every night. In doing this, you've created a training "split" that separates your training objectives into separate days. With the example just given, training each body area on its own day creates a six-day split.

But this is the real world, and we have to make adjustments. So the first step is to determine how many days per week you can fit in 30 to 60 minutes for training. It's probably not six days a week, and that's okay. If you have at least three days to focus on the training portion of your program, you will be doing just fine. If you have four or five days, that's even better. For the sake of being able to fully enjoy this program, I suggest doing everything you can to make the time to train at least four days. Regardless of whether you train three days a week or five days a week, you're going to be happier every single morning when you wake up from now on.

You might be wondering: If I can do it in three days, why train more? Think of your training routine like learning a new language. You're trying to grasp vocabulary, grammar, sentence structure, and so on. You can practice three days a week and get better, but if you spread that material out over five days instead, you'll retain more on each facet. That's what you're facing with fitness. You can work your chest and arms together if you have to, but you'll be able to put more emphasis on each muscle group if you have the option of training it alone. It doesn't mean one way doesn't work, it just means you might find it to be a bit better another way.

And if your regular routine has you training five days, but you can only train three days on a certain week, follow an adjusted split. Don't lapse a body part just because you're busy the day you normally workout.

An important part of selecting which muscles to train together and on which days to train them is ensuring you don't overlap muscle groups any more than possible. For example, you have to put a lot of biceps and triceps effort into training your back muscles just by nature of how the muscle contracts. As such, if you train your arms on Monday and try to train your back on Tuesday, you're going to find yourself at a disadvantage because of the soreness you might be experiencing. You won't be able to put full effort into your back training due to fatigued arms, and you'll also run the risk of overtraining your biceps and triceps. The solution is to spread them out, with at least a day in between; or in this case, and depending on the muscles and on your schedule, you might want to train them together. It's nearly impossible to avoid overlapping to some degree with certain muscles, like the arms, so just do the best you can to avoid training tired muscles.

Here are some suggested training areas for three-, four-, and five-day training routines:

Five days a week:

> Day 1: Chest
>
> Day 2: Back
>
> Day 3: Legs
>
> Day 4: Shoulders
>
> Day 5: Arms and Core

Four days a week:

> Day 1: Chest
>
> Day 2: Back and Core
>
> Day 3: Legs
>
> Day 4: Shoulders and Arms

Three days a week:

> Day 1: Back and Chest
>
> Day 2: Legs and Core
>
> Day 3: Shoulders and Arms

Days Off

You'll notice I don't suggest training seven days a week. That's too much. Remember that your body grows while you're at rest, not while you're exercising. As such, more isn't always better. That old adage was worn out the first time it was used.

When training properly, you should always have rest days. Use them as wisely as possible where your schedule permits. Try to space them evenly if possible or stagger them around what you consider your most exhausting body parts to train.

On a six-day split, the simple version is to train Monday, Tuesday, and Wednesday, take Thursday off, and train Friday, Saturday, and Sunday. You'll notice this will always result in six consecutive training days, but if you're only working a single muscle group, you should be able to ensure appropriate rest and recovery. And with that, if you have a muscle group that's particularly tiring—for me it's legs—train them before your rest day.

For a five-day split, you might go with a pattern like this: Training Day—Training Day—Day Off—Training Day—Training Day—Day Off—Training Day.

But, again, you have to do what fits your schedule to make sure you stick with the program. If you have to use a Train-Train-Train-Day Off-Day Off-Train-Train split, then it just comes down to being responsible enough to ensure adequate nutrition and sleep to make sure you recover.

Train Big Muscles First

On any days you're combining muscles, you want to train your bigger muscle group first. Even if you aren't training muscles that are directly targeted by other exercises, something has to give up a little bit of focus. As such, make it the smaller of the body parts. By training the bigger muscle group first, if another group is affected, it will act almost like an exercise of its own for that muscle as well. In contrast, if you focused on your smaller group first, you may find yourself too fatigued to put full effort into the bigger area. So if, for example, you're working your back and shoulders on the same day, train with your back exercises first. If you're training arms, train the triceps first (contrary to popular belief, the biceps aren't what makes big arms; the triceps constitute two thirds of the upper arm).

Volume Defined

"Volume" is a term used to define the amount of exercise you're doing. There is "exercise volume" (the total amount of accumulated work—sets and reps—on each separate exercise that you're doing), set volume (the number of repetitions per set), and total volume (the total number of exercises, sets, and repetitions you're conducting).

When you first start training, your volume should be relatively light duty, especially if you haven't trained before or it has been a long time. As you progress you'll be adding volume to the training of all muscle groups until a given point, which we will go over.

As you're building into your program, sheer training will create gains for you because your muscles will love the new stimulus you're giving them. You certainly will not continue adding volume forever, though (lest you find yourself training for hours and days on end), and in time can start employing a variety of techniques, rather than more sets, to keep your body growing. It's the same in professional sports. For example, in a sport like elite-level swimming, Michael Phelps doesn't just keep piling on the miles. His coach has found a *volume* that works for him, and within that volume, they've employed techniques with which they can keep improving.

Following are some volume suggestions for different periods of your training. The exercises and sets are strongly suggested, and the repetitions are a target. If you find you can do a few more reps, that's okay. If you find you can't get close, try an exercise that is easier to do, or use a variation of the exercise to make it more feasible. Remember, as you progress through your workouts you'll be doing different exercises and building general strength that will enable you to do more exercises later on. So don't worry if you can't do every exercise right now.

New Trainer Volume

As a new trainer, strive to get the following volume in your workouts:

Weeks 1–3: Two exercises per muscle group, three sets each, 15 to 20 repetitions per set

Weeks 4–7: Three exercises per muscle group, three sets each, 12 to 15 repetitions per set

Weeks 8–12 and beyond: Three to four exercises per muscle group broken up to a cumulative total of 9 to 14 sets, using a mix of 8 to 10 repetitions on more difficult movements and 12 to 15 reps for less intense exercises. For legs, stick with the higher range of the scale for sets and reps and go as high as 20 repetitions.

Throughout your training rotation, make sure you're switching up exercises every couple of weeks so that your muscles aren't getting used to the same movements week in and week out.

Advanced Techniques

If you feel your gains are getting a little stagnant, fear not. There are countless ways to keep things fresh. Here are a few ideas of techniques you can employ to ensure your continued progress.

Power Phases

Everyone has exercises that they find really, really difficult. We tend to avoid these movements because we don't feel we can do enough of them to make them count. And, in general, that's appropriate. You aren't a power lifter; you just want a great-looking body and to be healthy. But sometimes training like you're focusing on strength is good. So if the most challenging exercises for you are handstand presses or even one-leg squats, add in some of these exercises for a couple of weeks even if you can only get a few repetitions. You'll be amazed at how much you improve over time, as you build more strength.

These are called *power phases*, because due to the relatively few reps you're capable of, they focus more on building strength rather than visual muscle mass. But although strength isn't equally related to a lean body (look at power lifters and bodybuilders for contrast), there is a correlation between being able to move a larger amount of weight and continued progress toward your goals.

Increased Volume

At the opposite spectrum of the power-heavy phase, you can also throw in a short phase—a couple of weeks—in which you increase the volume—sets and reps—of all of your exercises. This too can shock your muscles into new growth.

Drop Sets

Drop sets are a method you can use to add extra intensity and create extra stress on your muscles. The simple explanation for a drop set is that you perform a set as usual, but immediately lower the weight you're using after you finish and start again. If you're using something like an adjustable dumbbell set, that makes it a seamless transition. But what if you're using body weight training principles? Out of luck, right? Nope. It's not a problem.

If you're training with body weight exercises, you simply adjust the tension or leverage you're using. This can mean changing from one version of an exercise to another, or just the angle you're using. For example:

Push-Up Drop Set |

> 10-reps push-ups with legs elevated
>
> Immediately switch to: 10-reps traditional push-up
>
> Immediately switch to: 10-reps push-up from knees

You can also do drop sets with squats and other exercises where you have the option of doing one-arm/one-leg versions.

Squat Drop Set |

> 10-reps one-leg squats (each leg)
>
> Immediately switch to: two-leg traditional squats

If you're feeling really adventurous, you can add …

Immediately switch to: Riding Stance for 30 seconds

You don't want to incorporate these types into every workout, because you can definitely sap your energy and tax your cardiovascular system. But if you hit a plateau, you'd be doing yourself a favor by throwing some drop sets in for a couple of weeks every other month or so.

Supersets

Supersets are similar to drop sets, in that there is constant motion. You go from one exercise right to the next, without stopping for rest in between. The difference is that instead of lowering the weight or resistance in/on the same exercise (like in drop sets), you're going from one full-on exercise into another. An example of a superset would be doing bent-over triceps extensions and going right into chair dips, or vice-versa. Pick two exercises that work the same muscle group, and do them back to back. Welcome to the world of supersetting!

Partial Reps

This term is largely borrowed from the world of bodybuilding where it is a very popular technique used to advance an athlete's training. Again, there's a common misconception that because it is a term derived from weight-bearing exercise it can't be taken advantage of by people who choose body weight training. Fortunately, as with drop sets, that is misleading. With a little care, you can definitely make use of partial reps. After doing as many repetitions as possible of an exercise using a full range of motion, start doing reps with as large of a range of motion as you safely can. For instance, if you're doing traditional push-ups, after you're too tired to do another full push-up, you may only be able to push yourself halfway up, which is a partial rep. You can do this with static and dynamic exercises.

On a biceps exercise, for example, you would go to full range of motion until you're no longer able to do so, then immediately switch to only extending your arms to the maximum distance in which you can still contract from. If it's push-ups, you simply would not bend your arms as far, which will allow you to still return to the top/starting position.

For exercises where you hold position, such as the Riding Stance for your legs, when you reach the point at which you can no longer hold the proper position, stand up slightly. You will be able to "ride out" the exercise for a bit longer.

"Partials," as they are often called, are a phenomenal way to ensure you're getting as much work out of your muscles as possible. Use them when you feel your training is closing in on a plateau and you'll notice yourself fly by that stagnant point with ease.

Forced Reps

Forced reps are most often conducted with a partner, but for exercises you're doing alone with a stretch cord or dumbbell, you can still put them to use.

The easiest example to use to describe forced reps is with a bench press. The athlete training would conduct as many full range of motion repetitions as possible on his own, and when he reaches the point where he can't return the weight to full extension, a partner helps just enough to get the weight returned to the starting point. But that isn't the end of the set. It continues until the partner is doing a majority of the work. This type of technique really helps create a burn in the muscle being trained.

Because the majority of people training with body weight routines train alone, forced reps are done a bit differently. They also must be practiced with care due to the body mechanics used.

With every exercise, perfect form is encouraged, isolating the muscle group being changed and using little to no motion from the rest of the body. But for advanced trainers, you can use just a slight bit of motion to help squeeze out some extra reps when you can no longer do so with perfect form.

Using a stretch cord curl as an example, when you can no longer reach full contract, bend at the knees slightly, and on the concentric portion of the rep right before you get to the "sticking" point you aren't able to get past, rock the body back just enough to finish the rep. A little "body english" is okay if done for the purpose of forced reps; just make sure it is never used when a strict rep can still be done, and always exercise caution.

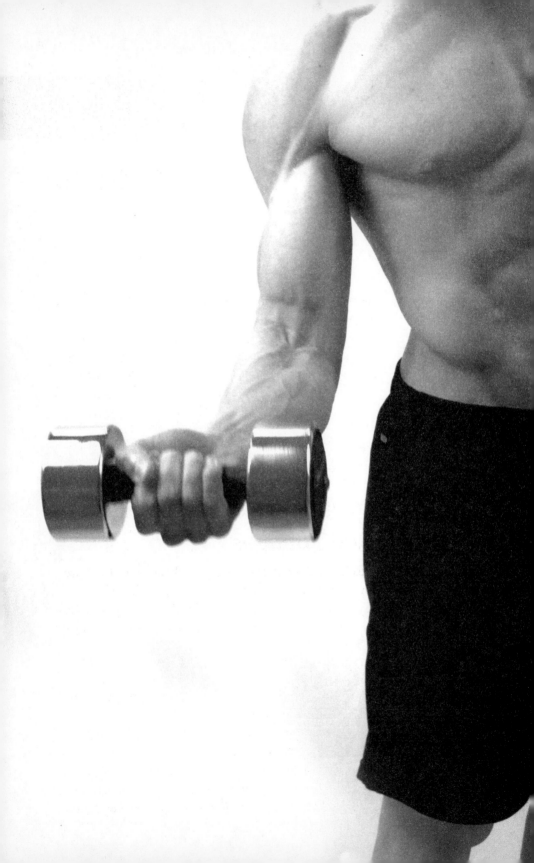

7

Workouts

By this point you're ready to get ripped. You know about proper nutrition, you know how to burn body fat, you know the proper form of cardiovascular exercise, you're trained in a myriad of exercises to grow every muscle in the body, and you're as close to an expert on stretching as you'll ever need to be. You know your schedule, and you have your routine time set aside. Now it's all about putting the ball in motion.

The following pages offer up routines that you can follow as is or mix-and-match to your own enjoyment. If you'd like to switch things out, just try to follow the volume that's laid out. If you don't like a cardio suggestion, change it up for something similar. Do what works for *you*.

Hand-Crafted Routines

The workouts that follow are set up for a 4-day workout split. If you are using a 5-day routine, simply break out the body parts needed to create the extra day. If you are in need of a 3-day split, then simply take the exercises from one of the 4-day routines and add them where they fit for you into the 3 remaining days.

You will notice on these workouts that everything is progressive, just as it should be for you. Start slowly and ease into your moves. Even the most gung-ho, hard-charging trainee-to-be can find himself crashing and losing all motivation if he pushes himself too hard at first. That's because this isn't just physical training; these workouts tax your nervous system, too. You have to be mindful of what your body is ready for. It's far better to start too slowly than it is to overdo it. If you've had some training background in the past and the first week or two of workouts that follow are too simple, go ahead and skip forward. But don't overdo it. Remember, this is a lifetime program, not something you can speed the results of by just doing more and more all at once.

With these workouts, the volume starts low because you don't need to do massive amounts of sets or reps to start seeing results. To give you an example, I had a bodybuilding client who had previously competed in high-level amateur shows. He was a big guy with years of hard training in his background and was very dedicated to his craft. But after taking a year off from training due to work commitments and welcoming his first child into the world, he wanted a new routine to get back into things. His first workout session focused on training his back. He did just four *intense* sets of pull-ups. Total. And he was sore for days!

These workouts start slowly with the training exercises. Then a little cardio gets mixed in. Then we pepper the workouts with a little more volume and a couple of twists. I also include some of the advanced techniques I described in Chapter 6. By the time you've done a couple of weeks of workouts included in these pages, you'll be a master at creating your own personalized routine.

No one knows your body like you, so listen to it, and if you find great results from something, even if it's unusual, by all means go with it. And most of all, have fun. You won't stick with the program if you aren't enjoying yourself, so make sure you're using the techniques you enjoy most, and don't be afraid to try new ones.

A final note: the repetitions listed here are merely suggestions. You might find you can't do as many in the early stages and then, after a few weeks, that you need more reps than written in these workouts to get a good workout. That's perfect! It means you're discovering your own limits and are getting in tune with your body. Don't take these numbers as mandatory; feel free to switch them up as you find necessary. Just try to follow the patterns. For instance, if you notice two sets have the same number of reps and the last set(s) have increased reps, try to do the same number of reps for *your* first two sets, and increase accordingly on your last set(s).

Additionally, if you have some sort of injury or experience any sort of pain while trying to do a particular exercise, don't hesitate to exchange it for another exercise contained in this book. There's plenty to choose from!

Week 1 Workouts

Day 1: Chest

Standard 7 Warm-up

Traditional Push-ups

> 4 Sets
>
> - Set 1 | 10 reps
>
> - Set 2 | 10 reps
>
> - Set 3 | 12 reps
>
> - Set 4 | 12 reps

Incline Push-ups

> 3 Sets
>
> - Set 1 | 10 reps
>
> - Set 2 | 10 reps
>
> - Set 3 | 10 reps

Day 2: Back and Core

Standard 7 Warm-up

Lifted Waves

>   3 Sets
>
>   - Set 1 | 10 reps
>
>   - Set 2 | 12 reps
>
>   - Set 3 | 15 reps

Cable Rows

>   3 Sets
>
>   - Set 1 | 10 reps
>
>   - Set 2 | 12 reps
>
>   - Set 3 | 15 reps

Push-up Hold

>   2 Sets
>
>   - Set 1 | Hold for 20 seconds
>
>   - Set 2 | Hold for 20 seconds

Side Planks

>   2 Sets each side
>
>   - Set 1 | Hold for 20 seconds
>
>   - Set 2 | Hold for 30 seconds

Day 3: Legs

Standard 7 Warm-up

Knee Drops

    3 Sets

    - Set 1 | 10 reps

    - Set 2 | 12 reps

    - Set 3 | 15 reps

Slow Stepping

    3 Sets

    - Set 1 | 15 reps

    - Set 2 | 15 reps

    - Set 3 | 20 reps

Wall Sits

    2 Sets

    - Set 1 | Hold for 30 seconds

    - Set 2 | Hold for 30 seconds

Day 4: Shoulders and Arms

Standard 7 Warm-up

Side Lateral Raises

> 3 Sets
>
> - Set 1 | 10 reps
>
> - Set 2 | 10 reps
>
> - Set 3 | 10 reps

Shrugs

> 3 Sets
>
> - Set 1 | 12 reps
>
> - Set 2 | 15 reps
>
> - Set 3 | 18 reps

Traditional Curls

> 3 Sets each arm
>
> - Set 1 | 8 reps
>
> - Set 2 | 8 reps
>
> - Set 3 | 10 reps

Triceps Dips

> 2 Sets
>
> - Set 1 | 10 reps
>
> - Set 2 | 10 reps

Cord Triceps Extensions

> 2 Sets
>
> - Set 1 | 10 reps
>
> - Set 2 | 10 reps

Week 2 Workouts

Day 1: Chest

Standard 7 Warm-up

Incline Push-ups

> 4 Sets
>
> - Set 1 | 10 reps
>
> - Set 2 | 12 reps
>
> - Set 3 | 12 reps
>
> - Set 4 | 15 reps

Decline Push-ups

> 3 Sets
>
> - Set 1 | 12 reps
>
> - Set 2 | 12 reps
>
> - Set 3 | 12 reps

Fat Blast Cardio: Walk for 2 minutes, jog for 30 seconds. Repeat six times.

Day 2: Back and Core

Standard 7 Warm-up

Cable Rows

>   3 Sets

>   - Set 1 | 10 reps

>   - Set 2 | 15 reps

>   - Set 3 | 20 reps

Ground Pull-ups

>   3 Sets

>   - Set 1 | 8 reps

>   - Set 2 | 10 reps

>   - Set 3 | 12 reps

Traditional Crunches

>   2 Sets

>   - Set 1 | 15 reps

>   - Set 2 | 20 reps

Abdominal Leg Raises

>   3 Sets

>   - Set 1 | 10 reps

>   - Set 2 | 15 reps

>   - Set 3 | 20 reps

Day 3: Legs

Standard 7 Warm-up

Wall Sits

> 3 Sets
>
> - Set 1 | Hold for 20 seconds
>
> - Set 2 | Hold for 30 seconds
>
> - Set 3 | Hold for 40 seconds

Single-Leg Straight Bends

> 4 Sets
>
> - Set 1 | 10 reps
>
> - Set 2 | 10 reps
>
> - Set 3 | 12 reps
>
> - Set 4 | 12 reps

Body Weight Squats

> 3 Sets
>
> - Set 1 | 10 reps
>
> - Set 2 | 15 reps
>
> - Set 3 | 20 reps

Fat Blast Cardio: Cardio Combination 1 (from Chapter 5)

Day 4: Shoulders and Arms

Standard 7 Warm-up

Cable Overhead Presses

   3 Sets

   - Set 1 | 10 reps

   - Set 2 | 12 reps

   - Set 3 | 15 reps

Side Lateral Raises

   3 Sets

   - Set 1 | 12 reps

   - Set 2 | 15 reps

   - Set 3 | 18 reps

Rear Laterals

   3 Sets

   - Set 1 | 10 reps

   - Set 2 | 10 reps

   - Set 3 | 15 reps

Cord Curls

   3 Sets

   - Set 1 | 10 reps

   - Set 2 | 12 reps

   - Set 3 | 15 reps

Doorknob Curls

   2 Sets

   - Set 1 | 12 reps

   - Set 2 | 15 reps

Triceps Dips

   2 Sets

   - Set 1 | 20 reps

   - Set 2 | 20 reps

Triceps Push-ups

   3 Sets

   - Set 1 | 15 reps

   - Set 2 | 20 reps

Week 3 Workouts

Day 1: Chest

Standard 7 Warm-up

Incline Push-ups

> 3 Sets
>
> - Set 1 | 10 reps
>
> - Set 2 | 12 reps
>
> - Set 3 | 15 reps

Platform Push-ups

> 3 Sets
>
> - Set 1 | 10 reps
>
> - Set 2 | 10 reps
>
> - Set 3 | 10 reps

Sliding Presses

> 2 Sets
>
> - Set 1 | 12 reps
>
> - Set 2 | 12 reps

Fat Blast Cardio: Walk for 2 minutes, jog for 1 minute. Repeat five times.

Day 2: Back and Core

Standard 7 Warm-up

Cable Rows

>   3 Sets
>
>   - Set 1 | 15 reps
>
>   - Set 2 | 20 reps
>
>   - Set 3 | 20 reps

One-Arm Rows

>   3 Sets
>
>   - Set 1 | 12 reps
>
>   - Set 2 | 15 reps
>
>   - Set 3 | 18 reps

Table Pull-ups

>   3 Sets
>
>   - Set 1 | 10 reps
>
>   - Set 2 | 12 reps
>
>   - Set 3 | 15 reps

Traditional Crunches

>   3 Sets
>
>   - Set 1 | 20 reps
>
>   - Set 2 | 20 reps
>
>   - Set 3 | 25 reps

Oblique Twists

>   2 Sets
>
>   - Set 1 | 15 reps
>
>   - Set 2 | 20 reps

Day 3: Legs

Standard 7 Warm-up	Riding Stances
Knee Drops	2 Sets

Standard 7 Warm-up

Knee Drops

   3 Sets

   - Set 1 | 15 reps

   - Set 2 | 15 reps

   - Set 3 | 15 reps

Front Kicks

   3 Sets

   - Set 1 | 8 reps

   - Set 2 | 10 reps

   - Set 3 | 12 reps

Hamstring Leg Raises

   3 Sets

   - Set 1 | 8 reps

   - Set 2 | 12 reps

   - Set 3 | 15 reps

Riding Stances

   2 Sets

   - Set 1 |
   Hold for 30 seconds

   - Set 2 |
   Hold for 30 seconds

Calf Raises

   4 Sets

   - Set 1 | 10 reps

   - Set 2 | 15 reps

   - Set 3 | 20 reps

   - Set 4 | 20 reps

Fat Blast Cardio: Cardio Combination 4 (from Chapter 5)

Day 4: Shoulders and Arms

Standard 7 Warm-up

Half-Over Presses

>   3 Sets
>
>   - Set 1 | 10 reps
>
>   - Set 2 | 10 reps
>
>   - Set 3 | 10 reps

Side Laterals

>   3 Sets
>
>   - Set 1 | 15 reps
>
>   - Set 2 | 15 reps
>
>   - Set 3 | 20 reps

Shrugs

>   4 Sets
>
>   - Set 1 | 15 reps
>
>   - Set 2 | 18 reps
>
>   - Set 3 | 20 reps
>
>   - Set 4 | 25 reps

Traditional Curls

>   4 Sets
>
>   - Set 1 | 12 reps
>
>   - Set 2 | 12 reps

>   - Set 3 | 15 reps
>
>   - Set 4 | 15 reps

Doorknob Curls

>   3 Sets
>
>   - Set 1 | 10 reps
>
>   - Set 2 | 12 reps
>
>   - Set 3 | 15 reps

Triceps Dips

>   3 Sets, Repeated twice
>   with the following pattern
>
>   - Set 1 | 15 reps
>
>   Take 10 seconds rest
>
>   - Set 2 | 15 reps
>
>   Take 10 seconds rest
>
>   - Set 3 | 15 reps

Cord Triceps Extensions

>   3 Sets
>
>   - Set 1 | 15 reps
>
>   - Set 2 | 18 reps
>
>   - Set 3 | 20 reps

Week 4 Workouts

Day 1: Chest

Standard 7 Warm-up

Platform Push-ups

>   3 Sets

>   - Set 1 | 10 reps

>   - Set 2 | 15 reps

>   - Set 3 | 15 reps

Incline Push-ups

>   2 Sets

>   - Set 1 | 15 reps

>   - Set 2 | 15 reps

Flyes

>   2 Sets

>   - Set 1 | 7 reps

>   - Set 2 | 9 reps

Sliding Presses

>   2 Sets

>   - Set 1 | 10 reps

>   - Set 2 | 10 reps

Fat Blast Cardio: Walk for 1 minute, jog for 1 minute. Repeat eight times.

Day 2: Back and Core

Standard 7 Warm-up

Table Pull-ups / Post Rows Superset

    5 Sets

    - Set 1 | 10 reps

    - Set 2 | 12 reps

    - Set 3 | 15 reps

    - Set 4 | 18 reps

    - Set 5 | 20 reps

Doorframe Pull-ups

    3 Sets

    - Set 1 | 6 reps

    - Set 2 | 8 reps

    - Set 3 | 10 reps

Elbow Holds

    3 Sets

    - Set 1 | 15 reps

    - Set 2 | 18 reps

    - Set 3 | 20 reps

Exercise Ball Crunches

    5 Sets

    - Set 1 | 15 reps

    - Set 2 | 15 reps

    - Set 3 | 20 reps

    - Set 4 | 20 reps

    - Set 5 | 25 reps

Fat Blast Cardio: Stair intervals. Find a flight of stairs and sprint up, touching each step, and walk down easy. Repeat for three rounds (up-down three times in a row), take a 1 minute rest, repeat four times.

Day 3: Legs

Standard 7 Warm-up

Hip Lifts

    4 Sets

    - Set 1 | 10 reps

    - Set 2 | 10 reps

    - Set 3 | 15 reps

    - Set 4 | 15 reps

Hamstring Leg Raises

    3 Sets

    - Set 1 | 10 reps

    - Set 2 | 12 reps

    - Set 3 | 15 reps

Rocking Push-ups

    2 Sets

    - Set 1 | 10 reps

    - Set 2 | 15 reps

Chair Squats

    3 Sets

    - Set 1 | 12 reps

    - Set 2 | 15 reps

    - Set 3 | 15 reps

Calf Raises

    5 Sets

    - Set 1 | 15 reps

    - Set 2 | 15 reps

    - Set 3 | 20 reps

    - Set 4 | 20 reps

    - Set 5 | 25 reps

Day 4: Shoulders and Arms

Standard 7 Warm-up

Half-Over Presses

    2 Sets

    - Set 1 | 10 reps

    - Set 2 | 15 reps

Cable Overhead Presses

    4 Sets

    - Set 1 | 12 reps

    - Set 2 | 12 reps

    - Set 3 | 15 reps

    - Set 4 | 15 reps

Front Laterals

    2 Sets

    - Set 1 | 12 reps

    - Set 2 | 12 reps

Side Laterals

    3 Sets

    - Set 1 | 12 reps

    - Set 2 | 15 reps

    - Set 3 | 15 reps

Cord Curls

    3 Sets

    - Set 1 | 15 reps

    - Set 2 | 15 reps

    - Set 3 | 18 reps

Towel Curls

    3 Sets

    - Set 1 | 10 reps

    - Set 2 | 12 reps

    - Set 3 | 15 reps

Triceps Dips

    3 Sets

    - Set 1 | 20 reps

    - Set 2 | 20 reps

    - Set 3 | 20 reps

Cord Triceps Extensions

    3 Sets

    - Set 1 | 12 reps

    - Set 2 | 15 reps

    - Set 3 | 18 reps

Triceps Extensions

    2 Sets

    - Set 1 | 15 reps

    - Set 2 | 15 reps

Fat Blast Cardio: Cardio Combination 2 (from Chapter 5)

Week 5 Workouts

Day 1: Chest

Standard 7 Warm-up

Platform Push-ups

> 2 Sets
>
> - Set 1 | 15 reps
>
> - Set 2 | 15 reps

Incline Push-ups

> 2 Sets
>
> - Set 1 | 20 reps
>
> - Set 2 | 20 reps

Decline Push-ups

> 4 Sets
>
> - Set 1 | 15 reps
>
> - Set 2 | 15 reps
>
> - Set 3 | 20 reps
>
> - Set 4 | 20 reps

Fat Blast Cardio: Walk 1 minute, jog 1 minute, walk 1 minute, sprint 15 seconds. Repeat four times.

Day 2: Back and Core

Standard 7 Warm-up

Cable Rows

　　3 Sets

　　- Set 1 | 10 reps

　　- Set 2 | 12 reps

　　- Set 3 | 15 reps

Doorframe Pull-ups / Ground Pull-ups Superset

　　3 Sets

　　- Set 1 | 10 reps

　　- Set 2 | 12 reps

　　- Set 3 | 15 reps

Knee-ups on Doorframe

　　3 Sets

　　- Set 1 | 10 reps

　　- Set 2 | 15 reps

　　- Set 3 | 20 reps

Side Planks

　　3 Sets

　　- Set 1 | Hold for 20 seconds

　　- Set 2 | Hold for 40 seconds

　　- Set 3 | Hold for 1 minute

Day 3: Legs

Standard 7 Warm-up

Slow Stepping

    2 Sets

      - Set 1 | 15 reps

      - Set 2 | 15 reps

Riding Stances

    3 Sets

      - Set 1 | Hold for 30 seconds

      - Set 2 | Hold for 45 seconds

      - Set 3 | Hold for 1 minute

Single-Leg Straight Bends

    3 Sets

      - Set 1 | 10 reps

      - Set 2 | 15 reps

      - Set 3 | 20 reps

Knee-High Jumps

    3 Sets

      - Set 1 | 10 reps

      - Set 2 | 10 reps

      - Set 3 | 10 reps

Calf Raises

    4 Sets

      - Set 1 | 20 reps, toes pointed out

      - Set 2 | 20 reps, toes pointed out

      - Set 3 | 20 reps, normal positioning

      - Set 4 | 20 reps, normal positioning

Fat Blast Cardio: Cardio Combination 4 (from Chapter 5)

Day 4: Shoulders and Arms

Standard 7 Warm-up

Overhead Presses

    4 Sets

    - Set 1 | 12 reps

    - Set 2 | 15 reps

    - Set 3 | 18 reps

    - Set 4 | 20 reps

Side Laterals

    2 Sets

    - Set 1 | 15 reps

    - Set 2 | 15 reps

Shrugs

    2 Sets

    - Set 1 | 15 reps

    - Set 2 | 18 reps

Shrugs to the Back

    2 Sets

    - Set 1 | 12 reps

    - Set 2 | 15 reps

Towel Curls

    2 Sets

    - Set 1 | 12 reps

    - Set 2 | 15 reps

Hammer Towel Curls

    3 Sets

    - Set 1 | 10 reps

    - Set 2 | 15 reps

    - Set 3 | 20 reps

Extended Curls

    3 Sets

    - Set 1 | 12 reps

    - Set 2 | 12 reps

    - Set 3 | 15 reps

Chair Dips

    3 Sets

    - Set 1 | 8 reps

    - Set 2 | 12 reps

    - Set 3 | 15 reps

Triceps Extensions

    2 Sets

    - Set 1 | 12 reps

    - Set 2 | 15 reps

Kickbacks

    3 Sets

    - Set 1 | 10 reps

    - Set 2 | 10 reps

    - Set 3 | 10 reps

Fat Blast Cardio: Continuous Punch/Kick combinations for 2 minutes, rest 1 minute. Repeat five times.

Week 6 Workouts

Day 1: Chest

Standard 7 Warm-up

Traditional Push-ups

      3 Sets

        - Set 1 | 10 reps

        - Set 2 | 15 reps

        - Set 3 | 20 reps

One-Arm Push-up from Knees

      3 Sets

        - Set 1 | 5 reps

        - Set 2 | 5 reps

        - Set 3 | 5 reps

Flyes

      3 Sets

        - Set 1 | 8 reps

        - Set 2 | 10 reps

        - Set 3 | 12 reps

Fat Blast Cardio: Jog 3 minutes, sprint 20 seconds, repeat four times.

Day 2: Back and Core

Standard 7 Warm-up

Post Rows

  4 Sets

  - Set 1 | 10 reps

  - Set 2 | 10 reps

  - Set 3 | 12 reps

  - Set 4 | 12 reps

Lifted Waves

  3 Sets

  - Set 1 | 15 reps

  - Set 2 | 20 reps

  - Set 3 | 25 reps

Doorframe Pull-ups

  3 Sets

  - Set 1 | 10 reps

  - Set 2 | 10 reps

  - Set 3 | 10 reps

Knee-ups on Doorframe

  3 Sets

  - Set 1 | 20 reps

  - Set 2 | 20 reps

  - Set 3 | 25 reps

Elbow Holds

  3 Sets

  - Set 1 | Hold for 40 seconds

  - Set 2 | Hold for 1 minute

  - Set 3 | Hold for 1 minute

Fat Blast Cardio: Choice of a Crawl/Sprint course (your choice of crawl exercises down a given distance, then sprint back to the starting point) of even lengths, 10 rounds. Start with 5 seconds rest and every other round, add 5 more seconds.

Day 3: Legs

Standard 7 Warm-up

Knee Drops

>   3 Sets
>
>   - Set 1 | 15 reps
>
>   - Set 2 | 20 reps
>
>   - Set 3 | 20 reps

Knee-High Jumps

>   3 Sets
>
>   - Set 1 | 10 reps
>
>   - Set 2 | 15 reps
>
>   - Set 3 | 20 reps

Exercise Ball Squats

>   4 Sets
>
>   - Set 1 | 10 reps
>
>   - Set 2 | 10 reps
>
>   - Set 3 | 12 reps
>
>   - Set 4 | 15 reps

Hamstring Leg Raises

>   4 Sets
>
>   - Set 1 | 10 reps
>
>   - Set 2 | 12 reps
>
>   - Set 3 | 15 reps
>
>   - Set 4 | 18 reps

Day 4: Shoulders and Arms Superset Workout

Standard 7 Warm-up

Side Laterals / Overhead Presses Superset

>   3 Sets
>
>   - Set 1 | As many as possible, both exercises
>
>   - Set 2 | As many as possible, both exercises
>
>   - Set 3 | As many as possible, both exercises

Overhead Presses / Rear Laterals Superset

>   4 Sets
>
>   - Set 1 | 10 reps / As many as possible
>
>   - Set 2 | 10 reps / As many as possible
>
>   - Set 3 | 10 reps / As many as possible
>
>   - Set 4 | 10 reps / As many as possible

Traditional Curls / Triceps Dips Superset

>   4 Sets
>
>   - Set 1 | 12 reps / As many as possible
>
>   - Set 2 | 12 reps / As many as possible
>
>   - Set 3 | As many as possible / 15 reps
>
>   - Set 4 | As many as possible / 15 reps

Triceps Extensions / Cord Curls Superset

>   4 Sets
>
>   - Set 1 | 10 reps / As many as possible
>
>   - Set 2 | As many as possible / 15 reps
>
>   - Set 3 | As many as possible, both exercises
>
>   - Set 4 | As many as possible, both exercises

Fat Blast Cardio: 10 Burpees followed by 1 minute of quick punch combinations. Take 30 seconds rest, repeat for five rounds.

Week 7 Workouts

Day 1: Chest

Standard 7 Warm-up

Decline Push-ups

> 2 Sets
>
> - Set 1 | 15 reps
>
> - Set 2 | 15 reps

One-Arm Push-up from Knees

> 3 Sets
>
> - Set 1 | 5 reps
>
> - Set 2 | 6 reps
>
> - Set 3 | 7 reps

Platform Push-ups

> 5 Sets
>
> - Set 1 | 10 reps
>
> - Set 2 | 10 reps
>
> - Set 3 | 12 reps
>
> - Set 4 | 12 reps
>
> - Set 5 | 15 reps

Fat Blast Cardio: Walk/jog easy for five minutes and focus on just high-intensity, challenging sprinting today. Follow this pattern: Sprint 10 seconds, rest 1 minute. Sprint 15 seconds, rest 50 seconds. Sprint 20 seconds, rest 40 seconds. Sprint 20 seconds, rest 30 seconds. Sprint 20 seconds, rest 40 seconds. Sprint 15 seconds, rest 50 seconds. Sprint 10 seconds, rest 1 minute.

Day 2: Back and Core

Standard 7 Warm-up

One-Arm Rows

   5 Sets

   - Set 1 | 10 reps

   - Set 2 | 12 reps

   - Set 3 | 15 reps

   - Set 4 | 15 reps

   - Set 5 | 20 reps

Table Pull-ups

   4 Sets

   - Set 1 | 6 reps

   - Set 2 | 8 reps

   - Set 3 | 10 reps

   - Set 4 | 12 reps

Doorframe Pull-ups

   2 Sets

   - Set 1 |
   As many as possible

   - Set 2 |
   As many as possible

Exercise Ball Crunches

   4 Sets

   - Set 1 | 20 reps

   - Set 2 | 20 reps

   - Set 3 | 30 reps

   - Set 4 | 30 reps

Flutter Kicking

   4 Sets

   - Set 1 | Hold 20 seconds

   - Set 2 | Hold 40 seconds

   - Set 3 | Hold 1 minute

   - Set 4 | Hold as long as
   possible

Day 3: Legs

Standard 7 Warm-up

Standing Rear Leg Extensions

>   2 Sets

>   - Set 1 | 10 reps

>   - Set 2 | 10 reps

Knee Drops

>   2 Sets

>   - Set 1 | 20 reps

>   - Set 2 | 20 reps

Static Superset

>   Riding Stance into Wall Sits

>   Hold Riding Stance for 1 minute, go into Wall Sit for 30 seconds

>   Repeat three times

V Dips

>   3 Sets

>   - Set 1 | 10 reps

>   - Set 2 | 15 reps

>   - Set 3 | 20 reps

Fat Blast Cardio: Stairs. Longer duration stairs today. Time yourself walking up and down stairs without stopping for 15 to 20 minutes.

Day 4: Shoulders and Arms

Standard 7 Warm-up

Overhead Presses / Shrugs Super-set

> 2 Sets
>
> - Set 1 | As many as possible, both sets
> - Set 2 | As many as possible, both sets

Side Laterals

> 4 Sets
>
> - Set 1 | 12 reps
> - Set 2 | 15 reps
> - Set 3 | 20 reps
> - Set 4 | 20 reps

Handstand Presses

> 2 Sets
>
> - Set 1 | As many as possible
> - Set 2 | As many as possible

Extended Curls

> 2 Sets
>
> - Set 1 | 15 reps
> - Set 2 | 20 reps

Hammer Towel Curls

> 4 Sets
>
> - Set 1 | 10 reps
> - Set 2 | 12 reps
> - Set 3 | 15 reps
> - Set 4 | As many as possible

Freeman Curls

> 2 Sets
>
> - Set 1 | 15 reps
> - Set 2 | 15 reps

Triceps Dips

> 3 Sets
>
> - Set 1 | 25 reps
>
> Rest 10 seconds
>
> - Set 2 | 25 reps
>
> Rest 10 seconds
>
> - Set 3 | 25 reps

Kickbacks

> 4 Sets
>
> - Set 1 | 10 reps
> - Set 2 | 10 reps
> - Set 3 | 12 reps
> - Set 4 | 15 reps

Triceps Extensions

> 2 Sets
>
> - Set 1 | 15 reps
> - Set 2 | 20 reps

Week 8 Workouts

Day 1: Chest

Standard 7 Warm-up

Traditional Push-ups

    2 Sets

      - Set 1 | 15 reps

      - Set 2 | 20 reps

One-Arm Push-ups

    2 Sets

      - Set 1 | 5 reps

      - Set 2 | 7 reps

Decline Push-ups / Incline Push-ups Superset

    4 Sets

      - Set 1 | 15 reps (Decline) / As many as possible (Incline)

      - Set 2 | 20 reps (Incline) / As many as possible (Decline)

      - Set 3 | 20 reps (Decline) / As many as possible (Incline)

      - Set 4 | 20 reps (Incline) / As many as possible (Decline)

Fat Blast Cardio: Cardio Combination 3 (from Chapter 5)

Day 2: Back and Core

Standard 7 Warm-up

Cable Rows

    2 Sets

    - Set 1 | 20 reps

    - Set 2 | 20 reps

Doorframe Pull-ups

    3 Sets

    - Set 1 | 4 reps

    - Set 2 | 6 reps

    - Set 3 | As many as possible

Table Pull-ups

    3 Sets

    - Set 1 | 8 reps

    - Set 2 | 12 reps

    - Set 3 | 15 reps

Lifted Waves

    4 Sets

    - Set 1 | 12 reps

    - Set 2 | 12 reps

    - Set 3 | 15 reps

    - Set 4 | 20 reps

V-ups

    3 Sets

    - Set 1 | 10 reps

    - Set 2 | 15 reps

    - Set 3 | 20 reps

Exercise Ball Ab Walk

    3 Sets

    - Set 1 | 10 reps (walking out and back in is one rep)

    - Set 2 | 10 reps

    - Set 3 | 15 reps

Fat Blast Cardio: Cardio Combination 2 (from Chapter 5)

Day 3: Legs

Standard 7 Warm-up

Cable Squats

> 4 Sets
>
> - Set 1 | 12 reps
>
> - Set 2 | 15 reps
>
> - Set 3 | 15 reps
>
> - Set 4 | 20 reps

Walking Lunges / Roman Deadlifts Superset

> 1 Set
>
> - Set 1 | Set up a course—a hallway or even in your own yard—and traverse it with lunges two to four times and have weights waiting for you when you finish. Immediately go into a burnout set of Roman Deadlifts.

Dumbbell Squats / Roman Deadlifts Superset

> 1 Set
>
> - Set 1 | 20 reps / As many as possible

Box Jumps Superset

> 3 Sets
>
> - Set 1 | 8 reps
>
> - Set 2 | 10 reps
>
> - Set 3 | 15 reps

Burnouts! Riding Stance / Wall Sits

> 4 Sets (Alternate Riding Stance and Wall Sits until you can't hold them any longer)

Day 4: Shoulders and Arms Superset Workout

Standard 7 Warm-up

Freeman Curls / Doorknob Curls Superset

> 3 Sets
>
> - Set 1 | 10 reps / 10 reps
>
> - Set 2 | 12 reps / 12 reps
>
> - Set 3 | 15 reps / As many as possible

Traditional Curls / Extended Curls Superset

> 3 Sets
>
> - Set 1 | 12 reps / 10 reps
>
> - Set 2 | 15 reps / 12 reps
>
> - Set 3 | 18 reps / As many as possible

Kickbacks / Triceps Dips Superset

> 3 Sets
>
> - Set 1 | 10 reps / 20 reps
>
> - Set 2 | 12 reps / 25 reps
>
> - Set 3 | 15 reps / As many as possible

Chair Dips / Cord Extensions Superset

> 3 Sets
>
> - Set 1 | 8 reps / 15 reps
>
> - Set 2 | 12 reps / 20 reps
>
> - Set 3 | 15 reps / As many as possible

Fat Blast Cardio: Cardio Combination 4 (from Chapter 5)

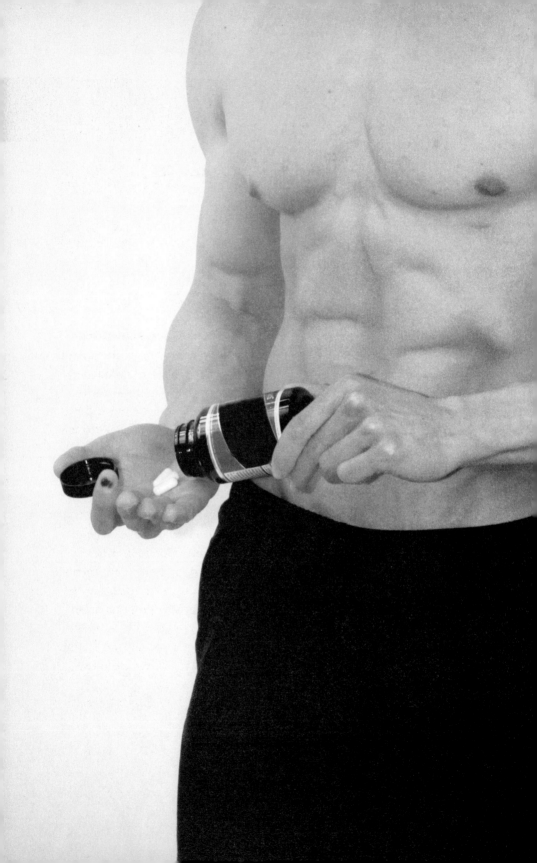

8

Beyond the Workouts

Nutritional Supplements

Billions of dollars each year are poured into the supplement industry. From manufacturers creating eye-catching advertisements to companies paying pretty faces and sculpted bodies to endorse products (which they usually have never used) to, ultimately, consumers paying huge mark-ups, it's big, big business. Often it's hard to see beyond the hype and find which, if any, supplements are actually worth their cost. In the end, a few really do have a place in a proper training program and, as luck would have it, some of the best are on the lower end of the cost scale.

The Truth About Supplements

No matter what you may have read in any of the major fitness magazines, and regardless of how sharp that guy on television looks when holding that fancy bottle of pills, you absolutely don't need supplements. There's a reason they are called "supplements" in the first place; they're ancillary, small additions that can complement a proper program. They aren't magic. Proper diets can give you all of the required vitamins and minerals you need. That said, if supplements interest you and are feasible for your schedule and budget, they can give you a little bit of an edge. But let it be stressed again, they are in no way mandatory. Never, under any circumstances, think it's acceptable to skip a good meal because you're taking a particular supplement.

Who Should Use Supplements?

Supplements can be safely enjoyed by a wide variety of exercise enthusiasts. There are, though, a few exceptions.

For the most part, people who are too young to have a grasp on proper training and nutrition should not use them. In general, it's largely dependent on maturation as to when the appropriate time would be to start a supplement program; kids of course simply develop at different rates. A lot can be gauged based on an individual's build at a certain age compared to peer median, training time, training level, and so on. And overall, that's the key to fitness and to athletic achievement, finding what's right for each person. Remember, nothing is one size fits all. As a general rule for parents, if you're worried about whether or not your child is mature enough for supplements, just go with the side of caution and wait. There certainly isn't any harm in not adding supplements to their diet.

You also shouldn't bother with supplements if you aren't willing to dedicate yourself to a steady workout program and eating properly. Simply by their nature, supplements are meant to be coupled with a program that is already giving the user results. If the training or diet isn't in line, vitamins merely create expense with no return.

Super Supplements

The simple fact is most supplements are junk, over-hyped, or over-hyped junk. You don't need the newest or "latest breaking supplementation breakthrough" to help you reach your fitness goals. A few of the basics will round out your regimen just fine.

Vitamin D

Most people don't get to enjoy year-round sunshine. For most, even when the sun is actually out, it's too cold to enjoy it for several months out of the year. As such, science has determined that a vast number of people have a deficiency in vitamin D (generally derived from skin exposure to sunshine). One great study that demonstrated this was done by the Australian Institute of Sport and looked into 18 athletes—female gymnasts aged 10 to 17—and found that almost all of them had vitamin D levels below recommendations.

Vitamin D is hugely important to the body. It helps treat and prevent a variety of diseases (including rickets, which is caused by its deficiency), and is known to aid in reducing everything from diabetes to obesity to arthritis. It also has been shown to boost the immune system, fight certain types of cancers, and increase energy levels.

Amino Acids

As we've discussed, amino acids are necessary for muscle and tissue regeneration and growth. Without repeating the discussion of the benefits of amino acids, they can be useful to people who are training, particularly those who are working to lose body fat. While you may be getting a variety of amino acids from your diet and through protein drinks, taking this supplement in liquid, powder, or capsule form can provide additional support for your lean body mass throughout the day without having to make a meal or mix a shake. Further, if you're dieting and trying to limit yourself to a certain amount of calories, a supplement is a very easy way to get your amino acids without adding a lot more calories into your diet.

Cinnamon

Most people definitely don't view cinnamon as a supplement (because it can be so tasty on a variety of foods), but if you don't have a taste for it, it definitely can be a viable part of your diet in pill form. Studies have shown that cinnamon can assist with blood glucose control in diabetes patients and also help prevent some types of cardiovascular disease. Some studies have even suggested that cinnamon helps boost cognitive function on a variety of tasks, including working memory and recognition abilities. There's also an added bonus: it's one of the cheapest capsule-form supplements on the market.

Multi-Vitamins and Minerals

Eating adequate amounts of fresh fruits and vegetables can be difficult even for the most dedicated of trainers. Your body needs a huge number of micronutrients and macronutrients for optimal health, and a quality multi-vitamin/multi-mineral is a great basic supplement to help get the body what it needs.

As with any supplement, you're going to want to make sure you find one that is of good quality. One way you can assist in this is to look for a bottle with the "GMP" stamp. This stands for Good Manufacturing Practices, which is an FDA standard that ensures a certain level of regulation, which is something that is, in general terms, missing in the supplement industry.

Men probably want to avoid using multi-vitamins with iron, while women should generally look for one that contains it. The reason for this is that although iron is essential to good health, too much in your body can be harmful. Very few adult men have iron deficiencies, which means it's much easier to end up with an overload of iron. Women, on the other hand, can benefit from supplemental iron as it is lost during normal body functions.

Whey Protein

Whey Protein comes in a number of forms and offers a huge variety of benefits. It can act as a great quick meal when needed, and helps easily increase the amount of quality protein in your diet. Protein helps reduce appetite and assists in muscle recovery and growth. A whey protein shake is the ideal way to complete a workout.

The best form of whey protein you'll find is isolate, which should be indicated on the label. Whey Protein Isolate is generally the highest quality of protein you can find and goes through the highest quality of filtering to remove unnecessary components. Percentage-wise, isolate has the highest amount of pure protein as compared to other whey types. It is the fastest-acting protein as well, which is what makes it most suitable for post-workout consumption.

Aside from Whey Protein Isolate, you will also find Whey Protein Concentrate in many supplements. This is a lower grade of protein, which contains less protein by volume, generally has added fillers, and is more slowly digested. Because it isn't as filtered as Whey Isolate, it does end up being significantly cheaper in some cases than the alternative.

To round out the options available in the whey protein market, you'll also find blends, which are combinations of isolate, concentrate, and other types of protein such as soy and egg. Given the available options, your best choices are those as close to Whey Protein Isolate as possible.

Creatine

When creatine first hit the market, there was a huge level of skepticism about its safety and effectiveness. Over the years, more and more studies have come out to show the effectiveness and the lack of side effects that accompany creatine use. Next to whey protein, it's likely the best cost-to-benefit ratio available on the market.

Creatine is a nutrient that is found naturally in the body and in foods such as red meat. When taken in supplemental form, creatine can assist in adding lean muscle mass, promoting physical recovery after exercise, and improving energy output. Furthermore, researchers have found that creatine has a protective effect from neurological disorders such as Parkinson's disease and Alzheimer's. More studies are necessary to really flesh out the full benefits of this supplement, but over the last decade, the evidence supporting its use has continued to grow.

If you're going to try creatine, stick with the basic and trusted form known as "creatine monohydrate."

Fat Burners

Fat burners are a huge market in the fitness industry. They get the biggest ads in the magazines and more "fat burning breakthroughs" hit the market every year than any other product. Some of these are beneficial to those who train hard, but likely not in the conventional way people think.

Products that claim to burn fat are generally stimulant-based, and most often this stimulant is caffeine. It's cheap, it's effective, and it does enhance exercise performance. But the actual "fat burning" effects are nominal. The actual increase in calories burned by taking these supplements are most often measured in the dozens of calories, not hundreds. These aren't going to give you washboard abs in a weekend.

These products do give you more energy to push harder during your workout or help you ease into longer-duration cardiovascular exercise. Again, it's a supplement, so you shouldn't expect huge jumps in performance by taking one, but if you find one you like and note an increase in mood or exercise intensity, go for it. But if you don't feel a difference from taking one, don't waste your effort or money.

Capsules, Tablets, or Liquids?

Whenever possible, purchase your supplements in capsule form. They maintain the integrity of the ingredient(s) better and are more easily digested than tablets. As for liquids, depending on the contents, you have to be particular about the temperature you store them at; improper storage can decrease their benefits.

Goal-Specific Supplements

Look at the shelves of any supermarket or supplement store and you will find a world full of fancy names that look like alphabet soup and flashy packaging. Here we help identify several supplements with known health benefits.

Improving Heart Health

CoEnzyme Q-10. Also known simply as CoQ10, studies have shown that this popular supplement protects the heart against oxidative stress. It has also been shown as a beneficial aid to slow the functional decline of Parkinson's disease among other conditions.

Improving Liver Health

Silymarin (Milk Thistle). Silymarin has been used for many years to treat liver conditions and to protect the liver. Studies have backed up its healthy benefits for the liver time and time again and even shown that Silymarin supplementation reduced the mortality rate of patients already diagnosed with cirrhosis of the liver.

Controlling Cholesterol

EPA/DHA. This combination of omega-3 fatty acids has been shown to lower triglyceride levels by as much as 30 percent.

Red yeast rice. This supplement has been shown to reduce total cholesterol concentrations, reducing LDL and triglyceride levels in supplement users.

Recovery

Your post-workout recovery is when your body gets the chance to put together new lean tissue and repair the damage (the good kind) done as a result of a quality workout. In addition to your nutrition, you should consider a few other factors to help get the most value out of your recovery time.

The Importance of Sleep

Sleep is paramount in the world of fitness. The less-than-glamorous truth is your body doesn't get leaner or stronger when you're working out, but only when you're resting. Particularly, when you're sleeping. And not getting enough rest has its own downside in addition to feeling lethargic and having diminished workout capacity.

A lack of sleep has been shown to predispose men and women alike to weight gain. A 2010 study published in the *Annals of Internal Medicine* showed a 25 percent decrease in fat loss in people who were sleep deprived. Further, short sleep duration in children has been shown to consistently correlate to future obesity. The take-home message is that quality sleep, for children and adults, is profoundly beneficial.

No amount of supplements will fix a problem derived from lack of recuperation. If you're getting less than six hours of sleep per night, you're at a much higher risk of suffering some negative effects not just on your metabolism, but also your mental focus and energy levels.

Consistency

Once you start your fitness program, it's important to stick with it. Don't avoid working out because your muscles are sore. The soreness will decrease over time as your body adapts. Also keep in mind that soreness isn't necessarily an indicator of a great workout, so as you're less and less sore over time, it means that you're enjoying the benefits of adaptation. As this happens, you'll be able to increase the volume and variety of training and, in the end, reap more benefits from your workouts. But consistency is key, so to enjoy these upsides, you have to make sure you stick with the program.

Understanding Overtraining

Training hard is great, but training beyond what your body can handle is an entirely different story. Doing so can suppress your immune system, cause extreme fatigue, and actually cause you to lose some of the gains you've worked so hard for.

If you find that you're mentally dreading working out, it's possible that you've been working too hard or haven't been able to take enough rest. If you wake up in the morning with an increased heart rate, this is another sign you may be overtraining. Take a day off, sleep in, and eat more. Get yourself back in the game, and then focus on balancing your training and getting enough rest.

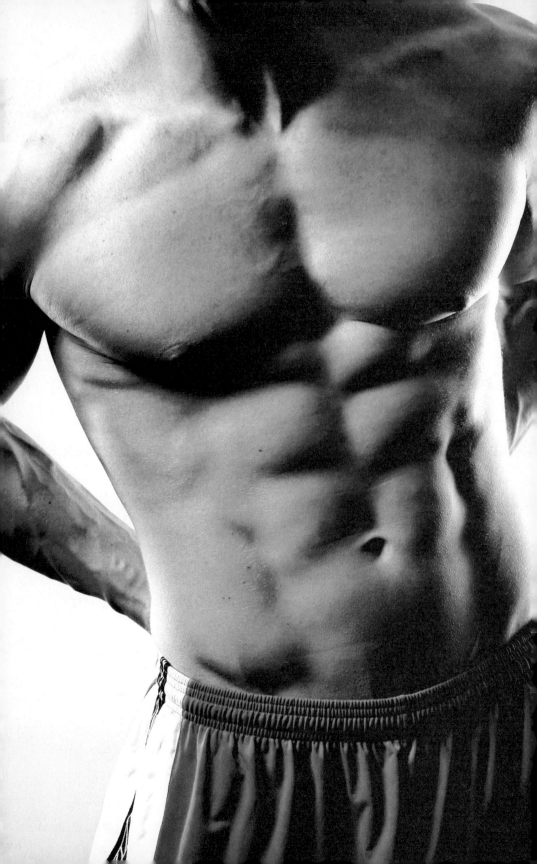

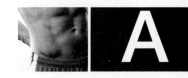

Glossary

aerobic   Any activity with the presence of oxygen. In fitness, any long-duration, sustainable cardiovascular exercise.

amino acid   The building blocks from which proteins are made.

anaerobic   Activity without the use of oxygen; for fitness purposes, refers to high-intensity, short-duration exercise.

BOSU   Stands for "both sides up" and refers to a popular training tool in which a flat platform is topped with an unstable rubber surface. Used for balancing and core exercises.

casein   A type of protein derived from milk that is slower to digest in the human body than whey protein.

CoQ10   Coenzyme Q-10, also known as Ubiquinone, a popular nutritional supplement shown to improve cardiovascular health.

creatine   An amino acid that encourages the body to store extra energy in muscles.

drop set   A continuous set of exercises in which the weight of an exercise is lowered after the first set with the goal of being able to conduct more repetitions.

EPOC   Excess Post-exercise Oxygen Consumption, referring to the amount of work the body continues to do after training in order to return to baseline levels of adenosine triphosphate (ATP) and lactate.

fitness ball   Large, round, ball-shaped equipment used as a platform for a variety of fitness purposes including weight training and stretching.

forced rep   A training repetition that could not be completed alone using strict form by the person exercising; often conducted with the help of a partner or body movement.

glycemic index   A ranking system for carbohydrates that refers to the speed at which they are converted into glucose and their effect on blood-sugar levels. The index runs from 0 to 100, with pure glucose having a GI of 100. Foods with a GI under 55 are considered "Low GI" while foods with an index ranking of 70 or above are considered "High GI."

HDL cholesterol   High-density lipoprotein, sometimes called the "good cholesterol."

hydrogenated oil   See *trans fat*.

LDL cholesterol   Low-density lipoprotein; often referred to as the "bad cholesterol."

metabolism   The total energy burned by the body to maintain homeostasis and normal function.

overtraining   A state in which the body cannot recover to baseline hormone and lactate levels due to an increase in training stress.

partial rep   Partial repetitions done at the end of a set after the person exercising can no longer complete full range of motion repetitions.

PNF   Proprioceptive Neuromuscular Facilitation; an advanced form of stretching that involves both stretching and contracting the targeted muscle(s).

recovery   The process of the body resting and receiving adequate nutrition and sleep to allow for the repair and growth of muscle fibers after working out.

serving size   The suggested portion size of a food; does not usually refer to all of the contents inside a container.

split   In fitness, the training routine defining exercise and rest days.

static   Exercises that are done by holding a fixed position; not moving.

stretch cord   A cord generally constructed of rubber that is used for a variety of fitness purposes, allowing the user to target muscle groups for training.

superset   Two exercises targeting the same muscle or muscle group(s) conducted back-to-back without pausing for rest in between.

trans fat   A polyunsaturated fatty acid created by the process of hydrogenation; trans fats are very difficult for the body to process.

volume   The total sum of training.

warm-up   A process of going through slow, easy motions to allow the muscles of the body to prepare for more intense exercises.

whey   A milk-derived protein that is popular among workout enthusiasts for the speed at which the body digests it, thus allowing for the quick uptake of amino acids. Most often used immediately post-exercise.

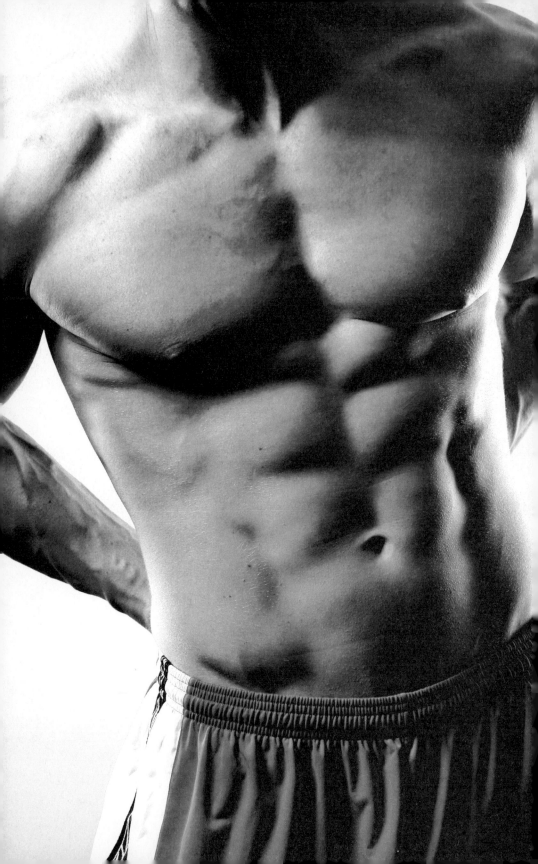

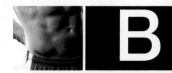

Sample Recipes for All Lifestyles

Healthy foods can be just as delicious as your favorite junk foods. The trick is all in the preparation. People who think that healthy eating is simply chicken and brown rice are stuck in ages long past. Included here are a variety of recipes, most very quick, very easy, and very delicious. And there's a little something for everyone here, no matter if you're a meat eater, vegetarian, or even vegan. Enjoy!

Easy Bites

Here are a few recipes that are especially beneficial when you need something quick or on the go. These are easy to put together and also make great travel mates. Unless noted, all recipes make one single serving.

Oatmeal Cookies

Cookies don't seem like they would have a place in a healthy nutrition program, but these healthier alternatives surely do. They offer quality carbohydrates for energy to keep you moving through your day.

Each serving (cookie) has:
80 calories
15 g carbohydrates
1g protein

---

2 cups whole-wheat flour	¾ cup sugar
2 cups quick oats	1 cup brown sugar
1 tsp. ground cinnamon	4 egg whites
1 tsp. baking soda	1 TB. vanilla extract
¼ tsp. salt	¼ cup fat-free milk
8 TB. unsalted butter	1½ cups chopped nuts

1. Preheat oven to 350°F. Spray baking sheet with non-stick cooking spray and set aside.

2. Combine flour, oats, cinnamon, baking soda, and salt.

3. Place butter in a separate bowl and mix until creamy. Add in sugars, egg whites, vanilla, and milk and mix until smooth. Slowly stir in flour mixture until blended, then add nuts.

4. Using a small spoon, portion dough 2" apart on coated baking sheet. Bake 10 to 12 minutes, or until cookies are lightly browned.

5. Transfer cookies to a baking sheet to cool completely.

Hard-Boiled Eggs

Eggs are nature's perfect protein. You don't always have time to do them scrambled or over easy, so try them hard-boiled and see how much more convenient these tasty treats can be.

Each serving has:
70 calories
0 g carbohydrates
7 g protein

---

1 or more eggs

1. Place egg(s) in a small pot and cover with water until water level is slightly above eggs. Bring water to a boil and, once reached, turn stove off, cover the pot, and allow to sit for 12 minutes.

2. After 12 minutes, pour the hot water out and immediately replace with cold water. Allow eggs to sit in cold water until cool, dump out water, and store eggs in the refrigerator.

Protein Pudding

This high-protein snack is a great alternative to sugar-laden puddings you see packaged on store shelves.

Each serving has:
210 calories
24 g carbohydrates
27 g protein

1 package sugar-free pudding mix   Protein powder
1½ cups skim milk

1. Make pudding as directed on packaging using the lesser amount of skim milk.

2. Once your pudding has reached its correct consistency, add protein powder to taste (depending on your protein choice, you may have to add more or less than you planned to achieve appropriate consistency).

Breakfast Yogurt Mix

You don't need a big breakfast to start your morning off right. Try this quick mix first thing out of bed and see how much better you feel as you head to work (or your workout)!

Each serving has:
300 calories
55 g carbohydrates
10 g protein

½ cup honey granola   1 cup fat-free yogurt
1 cup berries (choice)   (plain or flavored)

1. Combine honey, berries, and yogurt, and enjoy.

Beverages

Strawberry Banana Smoothie

You can also add a scoop of your favorite protein powder to this mix.

Each serving has:
250 calories
60 g carbohydrates
10 g protein

1 banana	8 oz. fat-free strawberry yogurt
2 cups strawberries (fresh or frozen)	1 cup fat-free milk (or soy milk)

1. Combine banana, strawberries, yogurt, and milk in blender and mix to desired consistency (add ice if necessary).

Greened Juice (Vegetarian)

This juice is packed with flavor and antioxidants.

3 to 4 kale leaves	2 to 3 celery stalks
1 medium cucumber	Small bunch parsley
2 cups fresh spinach	

1. Combine ingredients (in natural form) to taste and consistency into a juicer and mix. If necessary, add water to thin the juice.

Mocha Latte (Vegan)

A flavor-packed, healthy alternative to the mainstream mocha.

Each serving has:
219 calories
25 g carbohydrates
3 g protein

¼ cup organic fresh brewed coffee	1 tsp. raw Manuka honey
5 organic brasil nuts	¼ vanilla bean
2 tsp. sweet cacao nibs	Dash of cinnamon

1. Put coffee, nuts, cacao nibs, honey, inner seeds of vanilla bean, and cinnamon in blender or Vitamix and blend.

2. Add small amounts of boiling filtered water to reach desired consistency. (For a cold blended version, simply add ice before blending.)

Pre-workout Vegan Shakes

Option 1:

Each serving has:
520 calories
65 g carbohydrates
6 g protein

1 cup organic pineapple (skin removed)	2 TB. chia seeds
1 large leaf organic kale	½ cup organic raw shaved coconut
2 TB. maca	2 TB. coconut oil
	1 cup organic orange juice

Option 2:

Each serving has:
480 calories
60 g carbohydrates
4 g protein

---

1 medium organic beet	2 TB. hemp seed
1 small organic apple	2 TB. flax oil
1 stalk organic celery	1 TB. blue-green algae
1 large organic kale leaf	1 cup organic apple juice
2 TB. maca	

1. Put all ingredients in a blender or Vitamix and blend.

Blueberry Smoothie

Blueberries are as good as you can ever get when it comes to powerful antioxidants, and this tasty shake provides plenty along with some lasting energy to replace any high-sugared energy drinks you might otherwise reach for.

Each serving has:
410 calories
70 g carbohydrates
16 g protein

---

2 cups blueberries (fresh or thawed)	6 oz. 1% milk
1 cup low-fat vanilla yogurt	1 TB. honey
	Ice cubes

1. Mix all ingredients into a blender along with a handful of ice cubes and blend. If mixture is thicker than your liking, add more ice cubes until desired consistency is reached.

Meals

The most complete ratio of nutrients you'll get in your day should come during your seated meals—which means you need to eat the right things. These recipes are a great start to complete nutrition.

Veggie Wrap (Vegetarian)

This is a great, well-rounded meal for vegetarians and other discerning eaters.

Each serving has:
380 calories
40 g carbohydrates
15 g protein

2 TB. hummus

¼ cup sprouts

½ cup lettuce, shredded

6 kalamata olives

½ small cucumber, sliced

¼ cup feta cheese

2 tsp. olive oil

Lemon juice, to taste

1 whole-wheat pita

Salt and pepper, to taste

1. Combine ingredients in whole-wheat pita.

Bean Burrito (Vegetarian)

You don't need meat to create a healthy burrito that packs a lot of flavor and energy.

Each serving has:
320 calories
40 g carbohydrates
13 g protein

1 whole-wheat tortilla (lard-free)	¼ cup choice of cheese, shredded
½ cup black beans, cooked	¼ cup lettuce, chopped or shredded
Salsa, to taste	

1. Combine ingredients in tortilla, roll up tortilla, and enjoy.

Egg and Cheese English Muffin

This sandwich packs protein and slow-burning carbohydrates with just enough fat to slow digestion and keep you running for hours.

Each serving has:
300 calories
30 g carbohydrates
22 g protein

2 whole eggs	1 whole-wheat English muffin, toasted
1 slice fat-free American cheese	

1. In a bowl, using a fork or whisk, completely blend eggs.

2. Preheat skillet over medium heat.

3. Add eggs and stir to scramble; cook until desired consistency.

4. Just before eggs are done, adjust them to center of pan and place cheese slice on top. Cover until cheese melts, then serve on toasted English muffin.

Tuna Mix

Tuna doesn't have to taste so fishy; this recipe lightens it up.

Each serving has:
250 calories
15 g carbohydrates
30 g protein

1 can tuna (in water)

2 TB. mayonnaise made with olive oil

2 TB. relish

10 whole-wheat crackers, crumbled

1. Drain tuna and place into a bowl.

2. Mix tuna with mayonnaise, relish, and crackers until completely blended. This is delicious eaten as is, or with a side of celery.

Grilled Chicken Salad

This salad provides everything from protein to important vitamins and minerals.

Each serving has:
360 calories
20 g carbohydrates
35 g protein

1 boneless, skinless chicken breast

2 TB. olive oil

3 cups greens/lettuce

2 oz. feta cheese

1 TB. red wine vinegar

Salt, to taste

Pepper, to taste

1. Pierce chicken breast several times on each side with the end of a fork. Brush with 1 TB. olive oil and place on preheated grill, cooking for 6 to 8 minutes each side, turning once during cooking.

2. Cut grilled chicken breast into bite-sized pieces and place atop greens.

3. Add cheese and then top off with remaining olive oil and vinegar as dressing and salt and pepper if desired.

Paprika Shrimp

Shrimp is great on its own, but that can get old. Adding a little spice gives you a whole new flavor to enjoy a protein-packed favorite.

Each serving has:
200 calories
8 g carbohydrates
30 g protein

2 TB. olive oil   2 TB. paprika
6 oz. shrimp

1. In a bowl combine oil, paprika, and shrimp and toss to coat

2. Preheat skillet and cook shrimp over medium heat until done, approximately 3 to 5 minutes.

Ground Turkey Nachos

Mexican food often gets a bad reputation due to many restaurants using fatty ground beef. Changing just a few things brings new life to this old favorite.

Each serving has:
500 calories
35 g carbohydrates
70 g protein

2 whole-wheat tortillas
2 TB. olive oil, if desired
8 oz. 99 percent fat-free ground turkey
Taco seasoning, to taste
2 TB. fat-free sour cream

2 TB. salsa
¼ cup fat-free cheddar cheese, shredded
½ cup lettuce, shredded
1 medium tomato, diced

1. Preheat oven to 400°F.

2. Cut tortillas into triangles, brushing lightly with olive oil if using, and place on baking sheet. Bake tortillas until crisp, about 10 minutes.

3. Cook ground turkey in a large skillet over medium heat, seasoning if desired with taco seasoning.

4. Add ground turkey to tortilla triangles and top with sour cream, salsa, lettuce, and tomatoes.

Grilled Dijon Chicken

Chicken on its own can taste bland; low-calorie additions can spice it up.

Each serving has:
275 calories
1 g carbohydrates
30 g protein

---

2 garlic cloves, crushed

1 TB. ginger, minced

1 TB. Dijon mustard

1¼ cups olive oil

1 TB. low-sodium soy sauce

6 boneless, skinless chicken breasts

Salt, to taste

Ground black pepper, to taste

1. Preheat grill to medium heat.

2. Combine garlic, ginger, mustard, olive oil, and soy sauce in small bowl.

3. Brush mixture over both sides of each chicken breast and marinate in refrigerator for at least 1 hour.

4. Place chicken on grill and cook on each side 6 to 8 minutes, turning once when halfway cooked.

Quinoa-Salmon mix

By mixing salmon with quinoa, you're giving yourself quality protein and carbohydrates at the same time.

Each serving has:
490 calories
51 g carbohydrates
47 g protein

2 TB. mayonnaise (made with olive oil)	¼ cup onion, chopped
1 TB. fat-free Italian salad dressing	¼ cup red pepper, chopped
¼ cup celery, chopped	½ cup cooked quinoa
	½ can canned salmon

1. In a medium bowl mix together mayonnaise, dressing, celery, onion, and pepper.

2. Stir in quinoa and salmon and combine.

Turkey Tenderloins

On its own, turkey may not have as much flavor as beef, but done right you'll wonder why you ever chose higher-calorie beef cuts over these tenderloins.

Each serving has:
175 calories
2 g carbohydrates
30 g protein

2 cups sliced onion	½ tsp. salt
1 tsp. garlic, crushed	½ tsp. ground black pepper
½ cup white wine	¼ TB. Tabasco
½ tsp. dried thyme leaves, crushed	½ tsp. sugar
	2½ lb. turkey breast tenderloins

1. In a large mixing bowl combine onion, garlic, wine, thyme, salt, pepper, Tabasco, and sugar.

2. Place turkey tenderloins in large Ziploc bag and then add mixture, leaving a cushion of air in the bag. Allow mixture to coat tenderloins and marinate for at least 4 hours in refrigerator.

3. When ready to cook, place tenderloins in coated baking dish and pour marinade over top. Roast at 325°F for 30 minutes, or until turkey is thoroughly cooked.

Pan Tilapia

Tilapia is a flavorful fish that is high in protein and lower in mercury than many other fish.

Each serving has:
300 calories
15–19 g carbohydrates
40 g protein

Olive oil, just enough to coat pan	Lemon juice, to taste
2 (4-oz.) tilapia fillets	Salt, to taste
2 TB. fish-fry seasonings	Pepper, to taste

1. Coat large skillet with olive oil and preheat over medium heat.

2. Rinse tilapia fillets with cool water and shake off excess liquid.

3. Sprinkle fish-fry seasoning onto fillets and rub on lightly by hand, brushing off excess (this prevents accumulation but allows the fish to pick up the seasoning's flavors).

4. Place fillets into pan to cook, turning over halfway through (about 4–5 minutes). Before removing from pan, add lemon juice and salt and pepper to taste.

Protein Pancakes

By adding a little protein, these pancakes make a nutritious meal any time of day.

Each serving has:
320 calories
14 g carbohydrates
30 g protein

---

3 egg whites

1 tsp. vanilla extract

2 TB. low-fat cottage cheese

⅓ cup oats

1 scoop vanilla-flavored protein powder

Sugar-free sweetener, to taste

1. In a medium bowl combine egg whites, vanilla, and cottage cheese and mix well.

2. Add in oats and protein powder along with sweetener until mixed to a batter consistency.

3. Cook in large skillet over medium heat, turning over midway through cooking, about 3 minutes, depending on desired consistency.

Greek Burger

This burger recipe provides healthy fats, is high in protein, and provides a great deal of flavor.

Each serving has:
530 calories
8 g carbohydrates
60g g protein

½ lb. extra lean ground beef, 95% lean

¼ cup feta cheese

¼ cup sliced olives

1 clove garlic, chopped

Salt, to taste

Pepper, to taste

1. In a medium bowl combine beef, cheese, olives, garlic, salt, and pepper.

2. Form mixture into a patty. Cook on grill or stovetop over medium heat until meat reaches desired level of doneness, flipping halfway through.

Shredded Chicken Wrap

Chicken is so versatile that you can flavor it in many ways and prepare it in many ways while retaining its great nutrient profile.

Each serving has:
440 calories
30 g carbohydrates
35 g protein

1 poached, baked, or grilled chicken breast, shredded

1 whole-wheat tortilla

¼ cup lettuce, to taste

2 TB. nonfat Caesar dressing

¼ cup fat-free shredded cheese

1. Place shredded chicken centered on tortilla and top with lettuce, cheese, and dressing.

Tuna Wrap

This is just another way to enjoy tuna, but without the salty flavor that puts some people off from this nutritious fish.

Each serving has:
375 calories
27 g carbohydrates
42 g protein

1 can chunk light canned tuna in water	1 medium green bell pepper, diced
1 TB. mayonnaise (made with olive oil)	¼ cup lettuce, shredded to taste
1 pickle, diced	½ cup mushrooms, sliced
	1 whole-wheat tortilla

1. In medium bowl, combine tuna, mayonnaise, pickle, peppers, lettuce, and mushroom.

2. Place mixture in tortilla, roll up, and enjoy.

Sweet Steak and Rice

This recipe provides a nearly equal proportion of quality carbohydrates and protein, and is so tasty you'll wonder how it can be good for you!

Each serving has:
360 calories
33 g carbohydrates
32 g protein

4 oz. thin-cut steak, grilled	2 TB. sweet and sour sauce
½ cup cooked brown rice	

1. Cut grilled steak into bite-sized pieces and stir into brown rice. Top with sauce and mix together.

Tempeh Burgers (Vegan)

It's a common misconception that vegan eating lacks protein; this tempeh recipe provides plenty of quality amino acids.

Each serving has:
250 calories
15 g carbohydrates
25 g protein

1 lb. tempeh	¼ cup pineapple juice
2 TB. white wine	1 TB. ginger, grated
2 cloves garlic, minced	½ tsp. white pepper
¼ cup soy sauce	Red pepper flakes, to taste

1. Cut tempeh into four even patties.

2. In a medium bowl mix wine, garlic, soy sauce, pineapple juice, ginger, white pepper, and red pepper flakes together to form a marinade.

3. Coat patties in marinade at least 15 minutes.

4. Grill on medium-high heat 4 to 5 minutes on each side, turning halfway through cooking.

Steak Stir-Fry

This is a restaurant-style dish that offers loads of vitamins, minerals, antioxidants, and muscle-building protein.

Each serving has:
365 calories
14 g carbohydrates
46 g protein

1 TB. olive oil

6 ounces flank steak or chicken breast, cut into small pieces

½ cup broccoli, chopped

½ cup asparagus, chopped

½ cup mushrooms, sliced

1 small onion, chopped

¼ tsp. dried thyme

½ cup brown rice, cooked

Salt, to taste

Pepper, to taste

1. Add olive oil to large pan over medium heat and cook steak or chicken for 6 to 8 minutes or until done. And broccoli, asparagus, mushrooms, onion, and thyme and sauté for another 3 minutes.

2. Combine with cooked brown rice.

3. Add salt and pepper, and mix well.

Organic Tomato Sauce (Vegan)

Tomato sauce is a versatile topping for meats and other dishes, and this recipe provides heaps of antioxidants for a litany of health benefits.

Each serving has:
100 calories
8 g carbohydrates
1 g protein

---

4 organic heirloom tomatoes or any variety fresh ripe tomatoes (quartered with seeds removed)

¼ organic roasted red pepper—seeds and stem removed and blackened in a wok

1 small carrot, chopped

¼ tsp. or more olive oil

1 tsp. organic oregano

1 tsp. chopped fresh organic basil

1 tsp. sea salt

¼ tsp. black pepper

2 TB. vegan butter

1. Slice the tomatoes into quarters; squeeze the seeds out into a small bowl and discard.

2. Place tomatoes, red pepper, carrot, olive oil, oregano, basil, salt, and black pepper into a Vitamix blender and blend until smooth.

3. Transfer mixture to a large sauce pan and heat over medium heat. Add the vegan butter and stir until it melts. Adjust olive oil, salt, and seasonings to taste. If sauce tastes mealy in texture, simply add more olive oil until it is smooth. For a twist, add toasted pine nuts or kalamata olives and capers for a puttanesca vibe.

Soft Taco

Here is a simple, tasty way to have a soft taco without the grease or guilt.

Each serving has:
255 calories
17 g carbohydrates
25 g protein

4 ounces 93% seasoned lean
   ground turkey
1 medium corn tortilla

2 TB. red or green Taco Sauce
4 small hot chili peppers, diced

1. Cook ground turkey in a pan. When done, drain any fat and add just enough water to create steam from the pan.

2. Set tortilla on top of turkey to warm until soft. (Corn tortillas, unlike flour, are susceptible to cracking if not warmed).

3. Spread taco sauce on tortilla.

4. Mix peppers into ground turkey and add mixture to the tortilla.

Turkey Potato

Combining turkey and a potato is a tasty and quick way to get your quality protein and carbohydrates in at the same time.

Each serving has:
300 calories
19 g carbohydrates
22 g protein

4 ounces 93% seasoned lean
   ground turkey

1 potato
2 TB. salsa

1. Cook turkey in pan and keep warm over low heat.

2. Poke a potato several times on top and bottom and microwave for 6–7 minutes, then let sit for 3–4 more minutes.

3. Open potato down the center with a fork or use a fork to crush potato open.

4. Add turkey and salsa.

Quick Combinations

Sometimes you're looking for something that's quick but packs a lot of energy and nutrition. Long gone are the days when the only fast food you can find is a McDonald's double cheeseburger or some sloppy burritos from a convenience store. Try these for some energy, protein, and lightning-fast preparation.

Eggs and Toast

This recipe gives you long-lasting carbohydrate energy paired with nature's finest protein source.

Each serving has:
350 calories
16–20 g carbohydrates
25 g protein

Olive oil, just enough to coat pan	1 piece whole-wheat bread, toasted
3 whole eggs	
1 egg white	

1. Coat pan with olive oil and place over medium heat.

2. Fry eggs until the yolks are only slightly runny and place atop toast. Eat like a sandwich or cut with a fork.

Cottage Cheese & Pineapple

Cottage cheese has a texture that can be daunting on its own. Adding fruit like pineapple changes the consistency and adds a bit of healthy sweetness.

Each serving has:
190 calories
15 g carbohydrates
15 g protein

½ cup 4 percent milk-fat cottage cheese   ½ cup pineapple chunks

1. Combine pineapple chunks into cottage cheese and stir until mixed.

Turkey & Salsa

Each serving has:
150 calories
15 g carbohydrates
28 g protein

4 oz. cooked ground turkey (99 percent fat-free)   Salsa to taste

1. Stir salsa into heated turkey and serve.

Chia Yogurt

This ultra-quick combination is a great way to help fight hunger on the go. Chia seeds can hold a great deal of water, so while working through your system they help you feel fuller longer, which is a great pairing to the slow-digesting milk protein in yogurt. Furthermore, chia seeds are an amazing source of fiber and omega-3 oils.

Each serving has:
240 calories
28 g carbohydrates
16 g protein

2 TB. chia seeds

1 6-oz. low-fat yogurt or flavored yogurt

1. Combine chia seeds into yogurt and stir well.

Cottage Chia

This is as easy as the Chia Yogurt previously listed, but it packs a higher amount of protein and a bit less sugar.

Each serving has:
340 calories
21 g carbohydrates
37 g protein

2 TB. chia seeds

1 cup 2% milkfat cottage cheese

1. Combine chia seeds into cottage cheese and stir well.

Peanut Butter Apple

When you're feeling a little run down, the antioxidants and lasting energy in this quick bite will help pick you right back up.

Each serving has:
300 calories
28 g carbohydrates
8 g protein

1 medium red delicious apple   2 TB. natural or organic peanut butter

1. Slice apple and spread peanut butter onto slices

Oatmeal Breakfast Options

Save money and excess sugar calories by making your own oatmeal. Here are some suggestions:

Option 1: Cook ½ cup oats with natural, unsweetened applesauce and, when finished, top off with cinnamon.

Option 2: Cook ½ cup oats with a touch of milk and vanilla protein powder and add your favorite fruit.

Option 3: Cook ½ cup oats with a serving of raisins and cinnamon to taste. You can also add a bit of sugar-free maple syrup.

Oatmeal contains 150 calories, 27 g of carbohydrates, 5 g of protein.

Tuna Quick-Mixes

Mix one can of chunk light or albacore tuna with any of the following for a quick protein-packed meal:

- Lemon juice and fresh ground pepper

- Dill, mustard, and chopped celery

- Salsa and chopped green chiles

- Fat-free Italian dressing and fresh ground pepper

Each can of chunk light tuna has:
190 calories
0 g carbohydrates
42 g protein

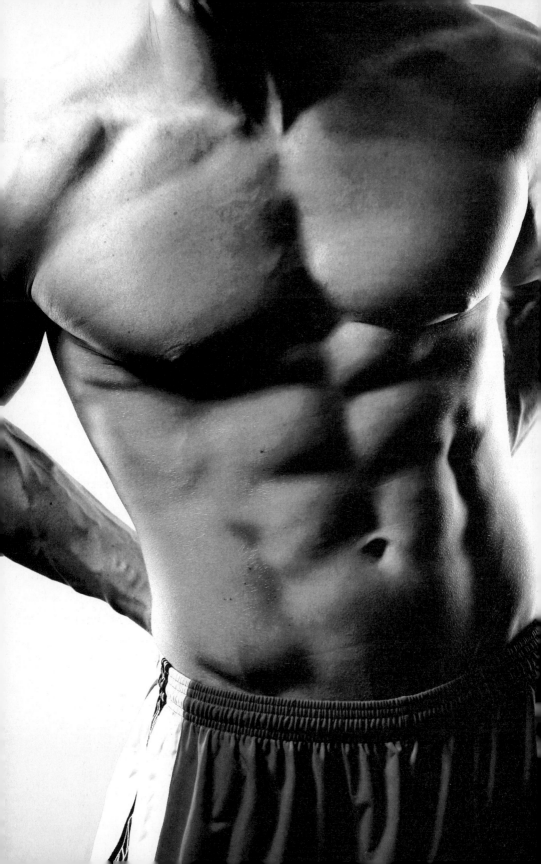

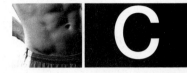

Contributor Bios

Rich Roll was named by *Men's Fitness* magazine as one of the "25 Fittest Guys in the World." He is a plant-based nutrition advocate and one of the world's top elite ultra-distance endurance athletes.

In 2010, Rich and another ultra-endurance athlete succeeded in the unprecedented *EPIC5*, which consisted of five iron-distance triathlons on five islands of Hawaii in just one week.

Rich is a 1989 graduate of Stanford University. He received his juris doctor from Cornell Law School in 1994 and is the founding partner in Independent Law Group, LLP.

Rich is also the author of the definitive plant-based whole food e-cookbook *Jai Seed*. You can learn more about Rich, his commitment to health, and his athletic endeavors at www.jai-lifestyle.com.

Megan Jendrick won two Olympic gold medals at the 2000 Sydney Olympics, winning the individual 100-meter breaststroke and swimming the breaststroke leg of the women's 400-meter medley relay. In 2008 at the Beijing Games, Megan took home a silver medal as part of the 400-meter medley relay.

Over the course of her career Megan has set over 30 American and World records and won 10 U.S. National Championships, 10 U.S. Open titles, 3 World University Games gold medals, and 2 World Championship silver medals.

Outside of her own competitive efforts, Megan is a model, motivational speaker, fitness columnist, and fitness author.

Paul Tomko is a graduate of the University of Washington and an NGA Professional Bodybuilder. Paul began as a competitive swimmer before changing his focus toward bodybuilding, and has competed around the country. He has won prestigious shows that include the Washington Ironman (Junior Division) and the NGA Grand Teton Invitational, winning the Heavyweight class and the Overall title to earn his professional status.

Index

hip exercises. *See* lower body exercises
hip lifts exercise, 104
hydrogenated oils, 33

I–J–K

incline push-ups, 69
ingredients, reading food labels, 33
interval sprints, 166

knee drop exercise, 93
knee lifts, 45
knee-high jumps exercise, 110
knee-ups on doorframe exercise, 116

L

lean stretch
  hamstrings, 147
  obliques, 143
leg exercises. *See* lower body exercises
lifted waves exercise, 84
logs (food), 15-17
lower body exercises, 90, 144
  bench stretch, 148
  box jumps, 109
  butterfly stretch, 149
  cable squats, 108
  calf raises, 112
  chair squats, 102
  cross stretch, 149
  fitness ball squats, 110
  floor stretch, 146
  forward lean stretch, 150
  front kicks, 101
  hamstring leg raises, 105
  hip lifts, 104
  knee drops, 93
  knee-high jumps, 110
  lean stretch, 147
  lunges, 92
  merry-go-round, 107
  one-leg calf raises, 113
  one-leg hip lifts, 105
  one-leg squats, 98
  rear extensions, 103
  reverse leg-ups, 106
  riding stance, 94
  rocking push-ups, 106
  roman deadlifts, 97
  side leg extensions, 104
  single-leg straight bends, 96
  slow stepping, 94
  squats, 91
  standing stretch, 145
  V-dips, 99
  wall sits, 100
  wall squats, 100
  wall stretch, 150
lunges, 92

M

manufacturer claims (food labels), 33-34
meal planning tips, 25-26
mental health benefits, 7-8
mental preparations, 5-6
merry-go-round exercise, 107
Milk Thistle, 224
minerals, nutritional supplements, 221-222

U

unconventional cardio exercises, 167-168

upper body exercises
    arms, 52-66
    back, 83-89
    chest, 67-74
    shoulders, 75-82
    stretches, 132-144

V

V dips, 99

V-ups exercise, 120

vitamins, nutritional supplements, 221-222

volume suggestions (training routines), 175-176

W–X–Y–Z

wall sits, 100

wall squats, 100

wall stretch
    back, 141
    calves, 150
    chest, 133

warm-up exercises, 44
    back squeeze, 46
    five-tier presses, 49-50
    five-tier squats, 47
    knee lifts, 45
    shoulder claps, 48
    slow bends, 45
    straight-arm circles, 49

water intake, benefits, 31

Week 1 Workout routine, 185-188

Week 2 Workout routine, 189-192

Week 3 Workout routine, 193-196

Week 4 Workout routine, 197-200

Week 5 Workout routine, 201-204

Week 6 Workout routine, 205-208

Week 7 Workout routine, 209-212

Week 8 Workout routine, 213-216

whey protein, 222-223
    concentrate, 38
    isolate, 38

weight loss considerations, 24

workout routines
    3/4/5-day splits, 171-173
    cardio training, 164-165
    drop sets method, 177-178
    forced reps, 179-180
    partial reps, 178-179
    post-workout recovery, 225-226
    power phases, 176
    rest periods, 173-174
    sample workout routines, 183-216
    supersets, 178
    volume suggestions, 175-176